Age Well!

A CLEVELAND CLINIC GUIDE

Robert Palmer, M.D., M.P.H.

with Eileen Beal

Cleveland Clinic Press

Cleveland, Ohio

Age Well!
A CLEVELAND CLINIC GUIDE

Cleveland Clinic Press

Contact:
Cleveland Clinic Press
9500 Euclid Avenue NA32
Cleveland, Ohio 44195
216-445-5547
delongk@ccf.org
www.clevelandclinicpress.org

This book is not intended to replace personal medical care and supervision; there is no substitute for the experience and information that your doctor can provide. Rather, it is our hope that this book will provide additional information to support understanding of the issues, conditions, and circumstances connected with the aging process.

Proper medical care always should be tailored to the individual patient. If you read something in this book that seems to conflict with your doctor's instructions, contact your doctor. Since each case is different, there will be good reasons for individual treatment to differ from the information presented in this book.

If you have questions about any treatment or practice mentioned in this book, consult your doctor.

The patient names and cases used in this book are composites drawn from several sources.

Library of Congress Cataloging-in-Publication Data

Palmer, Robert (Robert M.), 1946-
Age Well!: A Cleveland Clinic Guide / Robert Palmer, Eileen J. Beal.
p. cm.
ISBN 978-1-59624-042-1 (alk. paper)
1. Aging. 2. Aged--Health and hygiene. I. Beal, Eileen J., 1945- II.
Title.

RA777.6.P35 2007
613--dc22

2007007914

Cover Design: Whitney Campbell   Book Design: Ben Small, Joseph S. Kovach, Whitney Campbell

Contents

Introduction
A Road Map into the Future

I've been a geriatrician for twenty years. Like most geriatric doctors, I began my career as an internal medicine physician. I was drawn into geriatrics (a subspecialty of medicine that didn't even exist thirty years ago) by two things: my patients' needs and the needs of those caring for them.

The short definition of what I do is to coordinate the care of older people with serious medical conditions. The long definition would take up a telephone-book-sized textbook, like the two I've written or edited myself.

In fact, the idea for this book was born while I was working on *Clinics in Geriatric Medicine*, a text for geriatricians. It was a fun book to write – yes, fun – but I realized while I was putting it together that because it was written in *medicalese*, it would never be read by even one of my patients. Nor would it be read by those caring for someone at home who is elderly and disabled, or by middle-aged sons and daughters who hope to avoid the debilitating route into seniordom taken by their parents and grandparents.

Yet those people – the ones now in their late 60s and early 70s who want to age successfully, along with those in their mid-40s and early 50s who are the next generation down – are the ones I wanted to reach.

This book isn't intended to provide a magic bullet for optimal aging. (Optimal aging, by the way, has *nothing* to do with having wrinkle-free skin or an active libido as you sail into your 90s. It has *everything* to do with maintaining your ability to function and remain independent, mobile, and cognitively sound till then.) No such magic bullet exists. While you can fool the eye with plastic surgery and use a pacemaker to coax your heart into pumping like that of someone half your age, there's no such trickery with the brain or immune system. At 55 or 75 or 95, those systems are as healthy as your lifestyle habits and the mileage you've put on them have allowed them to be.

Think of your body as a car with many complex mechanical systems. No matter how much time you've spent washing, waxing, and polishing its exterior, if you've driven it hard, used poor-quality gas, and skimped on maintenance, it's worn out on the inside before it reaches the "classic" stage.

If you've been a careful driver, used the right fuel, and taken it in for regular oil changes and maintenance, it's still going strong at 200,000 miles.

So this book isn't about the mechanical devices (everything from pacemakers to ball joints) that you can install to make yourself feel younger or the exterior resculpting you can do to look younger (although if you follow the road map laid out here, you probably can do both). It's to show you that aging itself is not the cause of many age-related conditions. For instance, you can get gray hair anytime. It's just more likely that you'll get it at 50 than at 25. Ditto for bone and joint problems, wrinkles, and a host of other conditions that tend to come with advancing years. This book also will:

- Help you recognize the stages in aging: the young-old stage (65-74), the old-old stage (75-84), and the very old stage (85-plus), and teach you what to do before and during each stage to remain healthy, active, independent, mobile, and cognitively fit.

- Alert you to the landmarks for each stage of aging as well as the signs and symptoms, or red flags, for things that shouldn't be going wrong, so that you can seek proactive rather than reactive treatment.

- Show you why and how to change your expectations and goals over time to reflect the possibilities and challenges of each stage of the aging process.

- Give you the strategies, skills, information, and resources you'll need to create a lifelong optimal aging plan that uses lifestyle changes, health-care maintenance, and continuity of medical care to optimize the aging process.

- Clarify at what point in the aging process an older adult's care would benefit from a geriatrician's guidance.

- And, finally, provide an understanding of the biological, physiological, and psychological processes of aging, and enable you to set goals and make choices and decisions that reflect your values and desires.

Robert Palmer, M.D., M.P.H.
Head, Section of Geriatric Medicine
Department of General Internal Medicine
Cleveland Clinic

Chapter 1
The Biology of Aging

On August 4, 1997, Jeanne Calment of Arles, France, earned a spot in *The Guinness Book of Records*. After living 122 years, 5 months, and 14 days, the woman who had sold art supplies to Vincent van Gogh as a gangling 13-year-old, lived through two World Wars, taken up fencing at 85, bicycled around Arles till she was past 100,

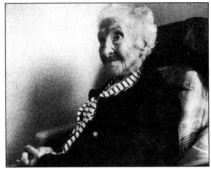

Jeanne Calment: The longest life span known.

and finally given up smoking when she was 120, died in her sleep at the nursing home where she'd lived for the previous twelve years.

Her death answered a major question: What is the absolute maximum life span for humans?

But it also left many questions unanswered. What is aging? Why do we age? Why do some of us age better than others? What's the optimal life expectancy for the rest of us? And most important of all, what can we do to maximize our chances of not just attaining that life expectancy but living healthily, actively, and independently till the end?

What do we mean by aging?

Aging is tricky to define.

It's *not* a condition like chickenpox, with definitive symptoms – a fever, oozing pustules that scab over, etc. It's a life arc of the interrelated and overlapping processes and changes in the body's 100 trillion or so cells that takes you from birth to death. Today in the United States, that arc, or expected life span, averages 74.8 years for men and 80.1 years for women.

Life span is only part of the definition of aging, though. For a true picture, you need to know the different kinds of aging arcs and which arc applies to you.

The suboptimal aging arc occurs when you're struck with major debilitating diseases or conditions early in life, don't have access to good nutrition or health care, and/or are living or working in an unhealthy environment, such as where everyone smokes or where groundwater is contaminated with lead. Under these conditions, it's a wonder you survive into old age at all. If you do survive, you're dealing with a high number of chronic and disabling conditions, and will probably spend two to four years in a nursing home.

Charting Your Biological Age

We age on two clocks: our chronological clock, which tells us how old we are in months, days, and years, and our biological clock, which, measuring against standard norms, tells us what physical "age" our body is.

To calculate your chronological versus your biological age, take the RealAge test at www.realage.com. Along with your "real age," the test calculates your body mass index and gives you a readout on how to improve your "score."

To take the test, you'll need current information on height, weight, blood pressure and cholesterol status, and the strength of the vitamin supplements you take.

In the normal aging arc, you put a minimum of time, effort, and energy into creating a strong, sound body to take into old age with you. Your idea of exercise is channel-surfing, you gave up milk for pop at 17, and have ignored your weight problem and risk factors for heart disease, arthritis, and other late-in-life chronic conditions. Your arc may be longer than that of the suboptimal ager, but it usually ends the same way: with chronic, debilitating conditions that result in a stay in the nursing home.

Finally, there's the optimal aging arc. If this is your arc, you've been front-loading on calcium and the other nutrients you'll need to draw on later in life. You've been proactive in addressing risk factors so they don't become medical conditions; you've been exercising regularly for the last twenty years; you gave up smoking in 1987, and you've been careful about eating red meat since 1999. Not only are your chances of aging well extremely good, but you're more likely to have fewer chronic diseases, compress them into a shorter period at the end of life, and spend little or no time in a nursing home.

There's nothing magical about optimal aging: If you hit the downward slope of the aging arc in better shape than the average person, you're going to complete it, barring accidents, well above the rest.

And if at your chronological age of 80 or 85 you have the strength, muscle tone, stamina, and vigor (your biological age) of someone five or ten years your junior, this will have a huge impact on your quality of life.

The stages of aging

Geriatricians break down aging into three distinct stages. Knowing what to expect at each stage can help you set goals for each one and plan for future care, including end-of-life care.

Ages 65-74: The young-old

If you've been taking care of yourself, this is a good decade because you aren't radically different from how you were in late middle age. However, this is a transition decade, characterized by changes in terms of function. You're at increased vulnerability for fractures and joint problems as well as for changes in nutrition status and energy and immune-system function. You take longer to recover after exertion, and diseases that you've managed to hold at bay begin breaking through your natural defense system.

For instance, if you've managed to escape type 2 diabetes, by the time you reach 70 you probably have it, not only because you've changed your exercise and eating habits, but because of the cell-level tissue destruction that occurred in arteries and capillaries in your 60s. When that happens, there is a cascading effect. You start getting hit with one disease after another: Vision worsens, blood pressure goes up, kidneys start losing function, erections become non-existent.

Hence, the focus for this age group is on disease prevention, screening, and the detection of diseases in early and treatable stages. Fitness priorities include weight loss for overweight patients, especially those with cardiovascular and/or diabetes risk factors, and a regular fitness program that includes cardiovascular and muscle-strengthening and toning workouts.

Bad as this sounds, there's an upside. We geriatricians used to talk about hitting the downhill slope at 40; then it was 50. Now we talk about 70. Maybe, by the end of this century, that's going to be 80 or 85.

Ages 75-84: The old-old

At this stage in the aging process, multisystem decline increases due to many things, including the cells' inability to repair themselves and the decline of the immune system. Since the body's defense system has been breached, most of the diseases and conditions that are going to affect you will indeed do so. And these diseases usually don't attack solo – they hit in clusters. Diabetes comes along with heart failure, and hearing loss or high blood pressure accompanies kidney disease and vision loss.

This cascade of conditions influences how aggressive diagnostic actions will be, how aggressive treatments will be, and the goals of therapy. Aggressive efforts are warranted for the treatment of chronic conditions – especially hypertension, coronary artery disease, and osteoporosis – and to prevent functional disability due to falls. However, at this stage, more consideration is given to quality -of-life issues, which are largely determined by mobility, function, and mental and cognitive state.

The key to having good quality of life in this stage is to have maintained good health long before you hit 75. If you didn't eat smart, get exercise, and treat and manage conditions that were modifiable early on (in other words, lay the proper groundwork for optimal aging), this is when and where payback starts.

Geri What?

Many people confuse geriatricians with gerontologists and vice versa.

A geriatrician treats the medical and psychological issues of aging; a gerontologist studies the issues of aging. While they are separate fields, the research being done by each group has a strong influence on the methods and practices of the other.

That doesn't mean that there aren't measures you can take when you're in your 70s and 80s to improve your health status (it's never too late to stop smoking or start exercising), but it does mean that no matter what you do at this point, if you haven't laid the groundwork, you're starting from a lower point on the health slope than if you'd been doing what needed to be done all along.

Ages 85 and up: The very old

When people live to be 85, they've definitely been doing lots of things right. So whatever they're doing physically, medically, nutritionally, emotionally, and socially, they should keep it up.

That said, due to the aging of organs, tissues, and joints as well as the cumulative effects of interacting chronic conditions, there is a tremendous amount of frailty and disability in those 85 and over. This means a more cautious approach needs to be taken with regard to testing and treating.

Preventive screenings and tests (such as mammograms, tissue biopsies, or blood tests) and aggressive interventions or treatments (such as a kidney transplant to "cure" kidney failure or chemo or radiation therapy to "cure" breast cancer) can be both physically and psychologically counterproductive. All decisions to use these kinds of interventions and therapies must weigh their short-term benefits against the rest-of-life discomforts or actual harm they can cause.

It bears repeating: How healthy and vibrant and vigorous you are at 85 or 90 is *always* going to depend on how healthy you were and how you worked to maintain your health at 55 and 65 and 75.

Why the body ages

To understand the effects of aging, it's important to understand the causes of aging. There are a number of theories about what causes us to age. Most fall into three groups:

Programmed aging

These theories focus on:

■ How longevity may be the result of the sequential switching on and off of a number of different genes that promote long life because they may protect the body against diseases at earlier stages in life. Or they provide protection to cells so that they stay hardier and healthier longer. Or they control or modify the biological conditions responsible for cell senescence and death. Indeed, those who are studying centenarians (those 100 and older) have found that they carry a gene (ApoE2) that the rest of the population seems to lack. Centenarians also tend to have had extremely good health all through their lives.

■ How cellular senescence, or the inability of cells to divide and replicate after between fifty and sixty replications, may cause radical changes in important cellular functions; how it may cause dysfunctional cells to accumulate in body tissues and organs; and how it may increase cell and tissue vulnerability to diseases associated with aging.

■ How biological aging may be connected with a biological clock unique to each individual that acts on the hormones of the endocrine system to propel, moderate, and control the pace of aging.

■ How immunological aging may be the result of an inevitable decline in the function of the immune system (especially of its fighter T-cells), which leads to increased vulnerability to disabling conditions (such as rheumatoid arthritis or shingles), infections (such as pneumonia), and diseases (such as cancer or Alzheimer's disease).

Aging due to wear and tear
These theories focus on:

■ How use of cells, tissues, and organs may lead to their wearing out.

■ How damage to cell DNA (everything from smoking to chemotherapy) may cause cells to go through negative changes (mutations) that accumulate over time, causing cell dysfunction, deterioration, and eventual death.

■ How free oxygen radicals circulating in the body may promote the production of a rustlike corrosive substance that damages and weakens cells and organs.

■ How the more an organism uses oxygen, which is usually a function of its size, the more its life span seems to shorten.

■ How the binding and accumulation of glucose (blood sugar) and proteins (composed of carbon, hydrogen, nitrogen, oxygen, and other elements), which is known as "crosslinking," may damage cells and tissues and lead to the slowing of bodily processes, or promote out-of-control cell proliferation.

Environmental aging

These theories focus on:

- How calorie restriction may influence both rate of aging and health status at each stage of aging. It definitely lengthens the lives of yeast and mice; the jury is still out on human beings.
- How at each stage of aging, lifestyle changes such as smoking cessation, improved exercise habits, and strict control of diabetes or high blood pressure may influence rate of aging and health status.

As you've probably noticed, all these theories are still in the "may" stage. Many are not mutually exclusive, and they are all about processes that are inevitable and immutable, and occur on several biological levels.

Deep-down results

It's easiest to see the results of the aging arc at the "macro" level, where they are clearly visible. You can see balding heads, wrinkled skin, cataract-filmed eyes and, with the help of an MRI, you even can see how the brain has shrunk. Other factors can cause these changes (including alopecia, radiation exposure, and Werner's syndrome), but in general, they are due to the process of aging.

The next level down is the "micro" level, inside the body where the organs are. Age-related changes to be seen at this level include a heart muscle that's enlarged or joint cartilage that's worn down to almost nothing. But in most instances, changes at this level can be seen only under a microscope or with the aid of laboratory tests, since they show up as changes in how the organs and tissues are functioning. Not even I, with thirty years of spotting abnormalities, can "see" that a person's liver isn't breaking down alcohol for excretion in the urine or that a patient's blood sugar is out of sight, though I can spot the symptoms of these situations.

At the submicroscopic level, age-related changes have an impact on how cells "communicate" with each other, take up nourishment and excrete waste products, promote biochemical and neurological reactions, and succeed or fail to fight off disease. It's at this level that most diseases and conditions of

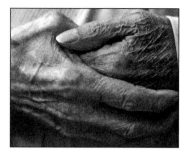

aging are born. For instance, it's at this level in the body's smallest vessels (its capillaries) that the tissue-destroying effects of diabetes first take place.

Age-related changes at the latter two levels throw up the red flags that propel people into the doctor's office.

Aging isn't maturation

While they seem like the same thing, biological aging is not the same as biological maturation. Maturation, which is mostly determined by your genes, is the process of tissue cells reaching their biological peak. After they reach maturation, they go into a plateau stage followed by a period of gradual and then, in some cases, precipitous decline.

It occurs at different times for different cell and organ tissues. Ovaries mature around the time puberty hits, at which time they contain about 2 million eggs (at death seventy years later, it's around 100); for kidneys, maturation is based on production of nephrons, which begin decreasing in number around age 30; brain maturation, on the other hand, is calculated by the number of new brain cells you make, and you stop making them at around 25; muscle reflexes and flexibility peak around 22, while muscle strength tends to peak around 30.

By the time you reach middle age, all your tissues, organs, and organ systems have "matured." From there, you're looking at a period of *relative* stability. But as each year goes by, the ability of those tissues and organs to maintain their normal function is increasingly threatened, and for the most part, the major threats are due to lifestyle. (More about that later.)

Aging isn't senescence

While aging leads to senescence – the organic process of growing older – it does not cause it per se.

Senescence, like maturation, is a segment of the arc of aging. Maturation, at the beginning of the arc, propels cells and tissues to the peak of their performance. Senescence, at the end of the arc, propels those same cells and tissues toward stasis, which for cells means decline, deterioration, and death.

I tend to think of senescence as the light bulb going out. The bulb works fine for thousands of hours, but all the while its filament, the part of the bulb that's actually producing light, is being stressed by being turned on and off, by the electrical charge it's carrying, and by white-hot heat. So it's changing. It's getting brittle, it's getting weaker, and it's becoming less able to actually carry the charge. One day you turn on the light and the bulb blinks out.

You think, hmm, the bulb just burned out, but in reality it's been burning out since the first time you turned it on. The last forty or fifty times you've flipped the switch, it's been a tossup whether it would go on or go out.

Outlook, expectations, and attitude

Up to this point, I've discussed mostly the physical and biological aspects of aging. But aging isn't just about what's going on in cells and organs; it's an emotional and psychological process, too. The better your psychological and emotional state, the more optimistic and outward-looking and positive you are as you age, the better your quality of life.

Quality of life, however, is in the eye of the beholder.

For example, take two 75-year-olds who have some vision loss and must use a cane to walk. One is bitter and angry and depressed, not just about the vision loss and the cane but about everything; the other, who may actually be a candidate for a wheelchair, is positive, optimistic, and outward-looking.

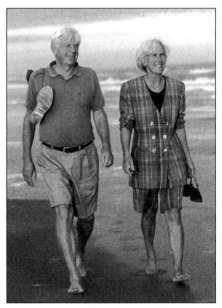

The former is going to see everything in negative terms – "I can't," "I won't," "I don't." He'll cut himself off from outside activities and create stress that's going to affect his blood pressure, put him at risk for a stroke, and lead to a poor quality of life. The latter is going to see things in positive terms – "I can," "I will," "I do." Because she is optimistic, has accepted and adapted to her limitations, and found strategies for maintaining cheerfulness, contacts, and function, she has created a life that is productive, rewarding, and satisfactory.

What Happens as We Age?

Aging is a one-way arc: You can slow it, but you can't stop it.

In your 40s, you begin to experience a series of changes signaling that you're on the downward side of the arc. Some can be modified; some can't. Your job – to paraphrase the Alcoholics Anonymous Serenity Prayer – is to modify the things you can, adjust to the things you can't, and have the wisdom to know the difference.

- Brain response time, reaction time, and recall (names, words, etc.) slow. By the time you reach your 80s, your brain weighs 7 to 10 percent less than it did when you were 25.
- Body composition changes (especially ratio of fat to muscle), requiring an adjustment in calorie intake and type (more fiber and high-quality protein, less fat), nutritional supplements (especially Vitamin B12, Vitamin D3, and calcium), increased water intake (due to decline in thirst perception), and exercise habits.
- Immune-system function declines, due in part to the shrinking of the thymus gland, which regulates the production of immune-system T-cells (fighter cells), leaving the body more at risk for infections, inflammatory diseases, and cancers.
- Eye lenses become less flexible, necessitating glasses. Long-term exposure to ultraviolet rays puts you at risk for glaucoma.
- Hearing loss (high frequency) begins around age 20; by the mid-60s, ability to hear low frequencies begins to wane. In addition, changes in the inner ear affect balance.
- Skin becomes thinner (due to the loss of underlying fat and collagen, which are rope-like strands that support the skin), drier (due to the loss of natural skin oils), and wrinkled (due to environmental exposure). In addition, hyperpigmentation (liver spots) begins to appear.
- Tactile sensation lessens, due to the normal effects of aging on the nervous system as well as dietary deficiencies and slowed circulation.

- Smell and taste decrease, due to a decline in the number of taste buds and olfactory nerves in the mouth and nose. This may lead to a decrease in appetite or increased use of salt to increase taste.
- The cardiovascular system is forced to work harder as arteries and heart muscles stiffen and become less flexible, due to aging and the accumulation of fatty deposits (plaque) inside arteries and veins. Circulation becomes less efficient, which impairs transportation of oxygen and nutrients.
- The lungs, chest wall, and diaphragm become less elastic. However, you only tend to notice this at high altitudes or when you're exercising.
- Gastrointestinal changes occur in the connective tissue and elasticity of the gut, causing digestion to slow and a decrease in the production of digestive enzymes. This can sometimes lead or predispose to malabsorption of vital nutrients (including calcium and the B vitamins), constipation, and gas.
- The liver takes longer to metabolize food nutrients, alcohol, and drugs (both legal and illegal), which may increase their potency and side effects.
- Kidney function declines, resulting in slower breakdown and clearing of toxins.
- Bone loss of about 1 percent a year begins around 40. Women may lose 5 to 20 percent of bone density after menopause, leading to an increased risk for fractures and/or osteoporosis, which is an equal-opportunity disabler: It tends to strike women in their 60s and men a decade later.
- Muscles lose mass, strength, and the ability to make quick recovery and repairs.
- Sex hormones decrease in both women and men, withdrawing their "protective" benefits. The functional activity of the ovary changes more with age than almost any other organ in the body.
- Irregular sleep patterns emerge, due to everything from the hot flashes of menopause to nocturnal trips to the bathroom, resulting in daytime fatigue, anxiety, and in some cases mild to moderate depression.

It's all about attitude

Over the past dozen years or so, studies have shown conclusively that positive mental health or a good attitude can influence physical health. They've also shown that certain personality traits such as optimism and pessimism, and being introverted or extroverted, can influence not only how well you live but how long you live well.

In fact, being an optimist may help reduce your risk of dying from heart disease and other causes. A Dutch study of 900 men and women ages 65 to 85 found that people who described themselves as being highly optimistic had lower rates of death from all causes and a 23 percent lower risk of cardio-vascular-related death than people who reported high levels of pessimism.

Pessimism isn't a risk factor just for dying before your time, however. The study noted that people who didn't have psychiatric problems but did have high pessimism scores on personality tests had a 30 percent increased risk of developing dementia several decades later. The same was true of individuals who scored very high on the test's depression scale. And the risk escalated to 40% or more for individuals who scored very high on scales for both anxiety and pessimism.

The study concluded that a predisposition toward optimism – seeing the glass as half full – not only seemed to enhance quality of life but provided a survival benefit, too.

Another study has shown the link between thinking "negatively" (brain activity was tracked in the right prefrontal cortex, a region linked to negative thoughts) and a weakened immune system, and how positive feelings can lead to reduced risk of death.

While it's not yet clear why or how things that clearly originate in the mind (such as enthusiasm, cheerfulness, and optimism) can promote longer life, it's clear that they do. And that's not all. Besides lowering the risk for early death, researchers have found that those who score high on being high on life also report:

- Fewer problems with daily activities, social activities, or work because of physical or emotional health
- Less chronic pain and fewer limitations due to pain
- Less interference from physical or emotional problems when they're engaging in social activities
- Increased energy
- Feeling happier, less stressed and anxious, and more peaceful and calm

By anyone's definition, that's quality of life.

Chapter 2
Prevention:
The Foundation for Aging Well

Both Maury G.'s grandfathers died of heart attacks in their 50s. So did three of his four uncles: two of his mother's brothers and one of his father's brothers. But Maury says that he didn't put "all those bad heart genes" into perspective until his father died of a massive heart attack at 57 in 1966.

"He was really overweight – Mom had been begging him to lose weight for years – and his blood pressure was over the moon," explains Maury. "He was chasing a kid, who'd been shoplifting, out of the shop they owned back in Philadelphia, and he didn't even get halfway down the block before he keeled over. By the time I got to the hospital the next day he was gone. I was a couple of weeks past my 30th birthday. My wife, Lil, and I had two boys and another baby on the way. I never knew either of my grandfathers, and now my own kids were never going to know my dad. I made a vow at Dad's funeral that I'd do whatever it took to be around for *my* grandkids.

"I got the first physical I'd had in years. And I told the doctor why I was there: I was scared, and I wanted to 'be there' for my grandkids. I left his office with a better understanding of how lifestyle changes could help me overcome my genes. I quit smoking. I cut down on salt. I joined our local

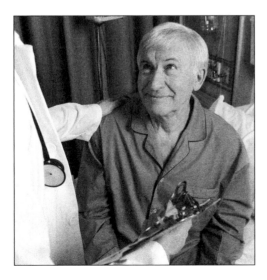

Jewish Community Center so I could swim a couple of times a week. And, when they put in an outdoor track the next year, I 'discovered' jogging. This was in the late '60s, so I was way ahead of the times on that."

But the smartest thing Maury and Lil did was start shopping at the local health-food store in the early '70s. "It was near the university where I was teaching,"

Maury says. "It wasn't so much what Lil and I bought there that turned us into healthy eaters, it was what we learned from the other people who shopped there. I bet half the residents from both the local hospitals shopped there, and a dietitian from the regional Veterans Administration Hospital did a monthly newsletter, including recipes, on healthy eating. One month it would be on food that was good for your heart – less fat, less salt, things like that. The next it would be on the foods that people with diabetes should be eating. Gradually, we totally changed the way we ate at home.

"I think our kids were the first ones on the block to eat yogurt and tofu," he adds with a chuckle.

And Maury's payback on forty years of keeping physically fit, eating "for life," seeing his doctor regularly, and managing his blood pressure and cholesterol with meds in order to keep heart attacks at bay?

At 70, Maury's not only *been around* for his grandkids, he's got the physique and stamina of a man ten years his junior.

Genes are not destiny

Genes are the life cards you're dealt at birth. Your lifestyle – what you do in your 40s, 50s, and 60s with the cards – determines how long and how well you will live in your 70s, 80s, and 90s.

A lot of hype about genes has been in the media recently, but despite what you've heard, genes are not the be-all and end-all of your existence.

They do help determine your longevity – how many years you will live. And they definitely set the stage for the diseases that you're predisposed to in old age. But they have no control over most of the lifestyle factors that turn a predisposition into a reality, and they don't determine how well you will age.

Lifestyle trumps genes

Genes don't control where you live or work. If your job or home puts you in close proximity to a factory belching smoke particles or chemicals that scour and scar your lungs, whether you're predisposed to lung disease or not, your life is going to be shorter and your quality of life worse because of your environment, not because of your genes.

Genes don't control your exposure to communicable diseases and injuries. If you waltz through life skipping your yearly flu shot and seldom fastening your seat belt, you increase your chances for life-threatening and life-shortening diseases and injuries.

Genes don't control what you eat. If you eat three squares a day based on the new USDA food chart, you get *all* the calories, vitamins, minerals, and nutrients you need for a sound, healthy body. If you don't, you end up undernourished or overweight, and dealing with the health problems that both conditions bring in their wake.

Genes don't control how much exercise you get. If you work out regularly, you keep your body in tiptop shape. If you're a couch potato, you put your body and health at risk for everything from obesity (which brings a whole set of chronic diseases and conditions in its wake) to Alzheimer's disease.

Genes don't control the preventive measures you take to maintain health. If you have every gene for longevity that's available and you've been smoking two packs a day since you hit puberty, the smoking will kill you long before the longevity genes say, "The party's over."

In other words, while genes *do* determine which diseases and conditions you are heir to, they become less "deterministic" as lifestyle behaviors begin to neutralize or heighten their impact. And they are doing that by the time you hit your 30s.

To paraphrase Dr. Tom Perls, author of *Living to 100*, if you want to be healthy at 60, 70, and 80, you'd better be taking care of yourself at 30, 40, and 50.

Prevention is the name of the game

To do that, you have to stave off as many of the preventable conditions and diseases as you can.

Prevention has three escalating goals. The first goal is to prevent the disease from occurring at all. If the disease does occur, the second goal is to prevent complications. And if the disease and complications progress, the third goal is to prevent them from causing irreversible damage. In medical terms, this is known as primary prevention, secondary prevention, and tertiary prevention.

For a good example of how prevention works on all three levels, look at what happens when you don't maintain a healthy weight.

Being overweight causes blood pressure to go up, and when it hits a certain point, you're diagnosed with hypertension. Hypertension can be controlled with medications, but if you don't take them, or take them erratically, you're at increased risk for stroke, heart attack, and heart failure, **and** your chance of developing kidney malfunction increases dramatically. If kidney function declines, that affects your ability to take hypertension (and other) medications. When you can't take the medications you need to control your blood pressure, the downward path you're on changes into the ski slope of heart failure, stroke, and/or kidney failure. With kidney failure comes the need for physically and emotionally stressful dialysis, or a kidney transplant. With a transplant comes the need for anti-rejection drugs that you'll need to take the rest of your life.

My point with this cautionary note is that stopping the weight problem upstream will solve all the problems that arise as a result of one very preventable condition.

How far upstream? One way to answer that is to say that by the time most of my patients come to me, I'm dealing with diseases that could have been identified with simple, usually noninvasive tests when they were *preexisting conditions*. Or they could have been treated at a much less advanced and therefore less destructive stage.

This is true whether I'm talking about cancer or cardiovascular disease or diabetes. When you detect, diagnose, and treat a preexisting condition or symptom early on, you don't treat a devastating disease later in life.

The multiplier effects

And you don't have to deal with what I call the "multiplier effect."

Let's use heart disease and diabetes as examples of how one "multiplier effect" works.

If you have only heart disease, its impact on you is "multiplied" by one: One disease, one impact. But if you have heart disease and diabetes (a very common "marriage"), your multiplier is two: Two times two equals four. That means that with the addition of the diabetes, your chance for having major complications with either or both conditions does not just double, it quadruples.

If you added another problem, say liver failure, your multiplier goes up to three: Three times three equals nine. That means that your chances for severe complications are nine times greater. Add another risk factor and … well, you get the picture.

But effects multiply, even when you have only one condition.

For instance, if you have diabetes and you don't get it under control, you get diabetes-associated complications. At first, only small blood vessels are affected. Since they reach every tissue in the body, however, soon every organ in the body is affected, leading to loss of heart muscle function, loss of vision, skin ulcers, gangrene, and the need for surgery. First it's a toe, then a foot, then a leg.

Diabetes is only one example. Left undiagnosed and untreated, kidney failure, heart failure, cancer, and dozens of other diseases cascade into the same kinds of irreversible complications.

And the more chronic diseases you carry into old age with you, the more vulnerable you are to both multiplier effects.

The pillars of prevention
(a.k.a. the nine habits of highly successful agers)

The good (no, make that great) news is that it's never too late to begin the prevention measures and strategies outlined in the following pages.

At their best, they can actually circumvent your genetic predisposition for certain diseases. For instance, if you have genes for high cholesterol, you're a candidate for a heart attack. However, if your physician put you on statins (cholesterol-lowering medication) the first time your tests went into the red zone, it's probably never going to happen. No matter how bad your genes are, statins lower cholesterol.

At their worst, these strategies can modify or diminish the impact the disease will have on your life, because no matter where you are on the life arc, the human body is incredibly adaptable.

1. Find a physician focused on prevention.
Once you hit your 50s, there's no such thing as a one-size-fits-all physician.

Physicians who focus on prevention will give you one-on-one consultations that create a doctor-patient partnership specifically geared to dealing with *your* medical and health circumstances, *your* life stage, and *your* health-care objectives.

You get *individualized* primary prevention because prevention-oriented physicians make sure you have all the immunizations, blood work, tests, and screens you should be getting to avoid diseases and disorders that threaten your health and independence. You get *individualized* secondary prevention because they diagnose and detect conditions and diseases in their earliest and therefore most treatable stages. And you get individualized tertiary prevention because they treat your conditions and your diseases appropriately.

It may be a bit more expensive to seek care with a prevention specialist, but payback is priceless. You're working with a partner, and you're ruling out diseases and/or catching them early enough for effective treatment.

Conditions and Diseases to Guard Against

Prevention is the key to good health as you age, but if you don't know the major problems to watch for, you may not be able to stop them at their earliest – and most treatable – stage.

Become familiar with the signs and symptoms of the following list of conditions and diseases most likely to affect those 65 and over:

Alcoholism	Influenza
Alzheimer's disease	Malnutrition
Breast cancer	Mild cognitive impairment
Cardiovascular disease	(often called pre-Alzheimer's)
Cervical/uterine cancer	Obesity
Chronic obstructive	Osteoarthritis
pulmonary disease (COPD)	Osteoporosis
Colon cancer	Pneumonia
Diabetes	Rheumatoid arthritis
Hearing loss	Skin cancer
Heart failure	Tetanus
Hypertension	Vascular disease
(high blood pressure)	Vision loss

2. Do a family medical "genealogy"

If you're in your 80s, climbing the family's medical tree isn't going to be of much benefit, but if you're 40 or 50, it's a good idea. Knowing your parents' and grandparents' medical history has great potential for guiding the tests, screenings, evaluations, scans, etc. from which you may benefit.

When a doctor knows a family history exists for a disease or condition, it puts the doctor on hyperalert and shapes the care offered a patient. For instance, if there's a history of skin cancers, skin screens will be done twice a year rather than once. Or if there's a history of colon cancer, the doctor will suggest a colonoscopy at 40, rather than the usual 50 or 55.

If you can't do a chart (easy-to-use charts are available for downloading on the Internet), then at least identify the diseases that have affected your "first-degree" relatives: your parents, brothers, and sisters.

And keep in mind that just because a disease turns up on your chart, it doesn't mean that the disease is going to turn up in you. The impact of your genes wanes as the effect of lifestyle behaviors waxes.

3. Get and stay physically active

Physical activity is the best medicine you can take (nutrition runs a close second). And it's never too late to start.

Studies show that no matter what your age or physical status, exercise improves muscle function, stamina, endurance, and strength; it helps reduce blood pressure and improves cardiovascular performance; it helps control diabetes; it promotes the production of all kinds of feel-good hormones (endorphins, serotonin, dopamine, adrenalin) so that you feel refreshed and vitalized (and not hungry) for hours afterward; it improves balance and gait; it burns calories so that you don't have to deprive yourself of food; and it costs as little (a $39 pair of walking shoes) or as much (a $1,000 health club membership) as you feel like paying. (Many clubs have senior discounts, by the way.)

Studies indicate that you don't have to engage in sustained exercise for a specified number of minutes or break out in a sweat for it to be effective. Five minutes here, ten minutes there, it all adds up. Studies also indicate that exercise may help "unload" more oxygen from red blood cells into the body's tissues to keep them better nourished. And studies show that people with major depression who participate in exercise programs have fewer depressive symptoms and require less medication. All these effects start to show results from the get-go. Once they begin, people who have not been exercising or who have never exercised experience benefits almost immediately.

4. Practice smart eating

As you move through each age stage (65-74, 75-84, over 85), the importance of diet and nutrition increases. Not only do your nutrition needs change, the way your body uses (metabolizes) the calories and nutrients you're taking in changes – and for the most part, the changes are on the negative side. Due to a decline in your "lean" muscle mass (the muscles used for strength and mobility) and an increase in your fat-to-muscle ratio, you need fewer calories for energy. Due to changes in the digestive tract, you aren't processing food as well as you used to, so it's important that the foods you take in be nutrient-dense. In other words, what you eat needs to be heavy on (or fortified with) vitamins, minerals, cell-building and -repairing amino acids and fatty acids, trace elements, fiber, etc., and it needs to be light on calories.

If you don't get the nutrients you need from your food, especially protein and calcium, your body will rob muscle and bone to get them. That means an increased risk for gait problems, falls, and broken bones.

Most nutrition problems can be addressed just by eating a well-balanced diet but, due to everything from tooth loss to depression, many older adults can't get the nutrients they need in the food they eat. When that occurs, vitamin-mineral and liquid supplements are a valid substitute for the real thing.

5. Achieve and maintain a healthy weight for your age

Weight is relative. What is healthy for someone at one stage of life may not be healthy for that person at a later stage. That said, if you were healthy at a certain weight at age 50, despite the muscle-to-fat shift that will have taken place, you should be healthy at or near that weight in your 70s and 80s.

Unfortunately, most people can't maintain a healthy weight just by eating smart. To maintain weight, you need to coordinate a smart eating program with a smart exercise program. And the earlier you do that, the better. If you develop an exercise habit early on and make a place for it in your daily schedule, it's easier to maintain the habit as you get older.

Charting the Family Medical History

If you know your heredity quotient (HQ) for a particular disease, you can usually take measures to prevent it or lessen its impact.

To find your HQ, start by using a standard genealogy chart (you can find and download free charts from the Internet) to make a detailed medical history of you and your family.

First, ask your physician for a rundown on which of your medical conditions, including addictions and mental illnesses, have a genetic link.

Then talk to parents, grandparents, and siblings about their health problems – chronic diseases, non-life-threatening disorders, things they are seeing their physician about – and the age they were when these problems seemed to kick in.

After you chart your HQ, start working on your prevention quotient (PQ), the effect behavior and lifestyle have on diseases and conditions. For some diseases, such as osteoarthritis or Huntington's disease, PQ is low; there is little you can do to prevent them. Others, such as diabetes or lung cancer, have a high PQ, meaning there's lots you can do to prevent them and lessen their impact if they do strike.

What's the best source of PQ info and strategies? Your doctor, who'll be able to provide you with information on the medical exams, screenings, and tests you should be doing on a regular basis and the lifestyle changes you should make to boost your PQ.

The next best sources of information are organizations, such as the American Cancer Society or American Diabetes Association, which deal specifically with the disease to which you are genetically disposed. Local chapters are listed in the telephone book; websites of national offices can be found on the Internet.

Another good source is www.rarediseases.org, the national organization for "orphan" disorders, diseases, and conditions.

6. Stay mentally active

As we age, brain function slows down. So do aspects like eye-hand coordination on the tennis court and eye-foot coordination in the car.

Studies show that people who engage in mentally and physically stimulating activities are less likely to develop dementia-related cognitive decline than those who don't stay mentally on the ball. And if their cognitive faculties should decline, they will do so more slowly.

Activities that keep the mind buzzing come in all forms and at all intellectual levels. Chess and word-search puzzles, discussion and book groups, visits to art galleries or museums, hikes through Civil War battlefields, classes on paper-cutting or orchid-breeding or jewelry-making, lessons in piano or computer or t'ai chi or the tango, a part-time job at the local nursery, or a week spent at an Elderhostel learning about the Indian cultures of the Southwest are all examples of cognitively stimulating, challenging, engaging, and rewarding activities.

Cognitively stimulating activities have another payoff. They tend to be socially and emotionally satisfying, too. Not only do they strengthen and maintain brain health and function, they strengthen and maintain mental health as well.

7. Boost emotional and psychological well-being

As you age, attitude is everything. Despite the fact that they may be dealing with the chronic pain of arthritis or the diet restrictions imposed by diabetes, people with a positive attitude are less stressed, feel less pain, and are more involved with family, friends, and a social network. In addition to the emotional benefits, they gain physical benefits as well. In general, those who see the glass as half full are more motivated to practice smart eating, exercise, take their medications, and go in for follow-up visits with their physicians.

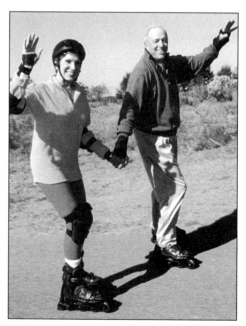

Staying positive creates a cascade of benefits that loop back on themselves to produce even better emotional, psychological, and physical health.

If those who tend to see the glass as half empty join support groups,

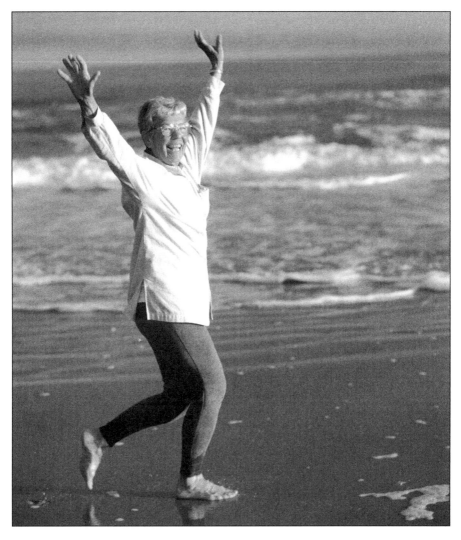

they may be able to develop strategies that mimic a positive attitude. Studies show that participation pays off handsomely in lowered stress and depression levels, better medication adherence and cognitive function, etc.

8. Stop tobacco use

Smoking has an impact on every organ system in your body. Smoking cessation is the single most important thing you can do to improve your health, lengthen your life, and improve your quality of life. Nothing exceeds the benefit you get if you stop smoking, and that benefit is both immediate and long-term.

And it's never too late to stop. You cannot regenerate scarred throat and lung tissue, but tissue that is not irreversibly damaged can and does regain function. And symptoms that remain – emphysema, bronchitis, arterial disease, etc. – can be treated more effectively with less medication.

9. Plan to age

You can age helter-skelter and meet every age-related health and function change in crisis mode, or you can plan for change the way you plan financially for retirement.

As with your financial planning, planning to age well isn't something you can do on your own. You need the counsel and advice of such experts as geriatricians, geriatric social workers, and occupational therapists – in other words, people who can help you map your future by asking you questions about how you want to live, where you want to live, the kind of home you want to live in, the activities you want to pursue at 70, 75, and 80, where you want to live when you can't take care of yourself, etc.

And waiting till you're 65 and walking out the office door for the last time is not the time to start your planning. It should be an evolutionary process initiated in your mid- to late-50s. If you take this approach, by the time you sail into retirement you've charted a course for the future and found the mechanisms, strategies, trade-offs, and substitutions that are going to help you get there in the best possible physical and emotional shape.

Chapter 3
Eating for Life

When her daughter brought the recently widowed 82-year-old Leda S. to my office, I knew immediately why she was there. I'd seen Leda a few months before, and between her last visit and this one she'd lost a lot of weight – nine and a half pounds, as it turned out.

Since I knew the family, I suspected the reason for the weight loss, but I still did a basic physical, a blood panel (to check calcium, iron, and vitamin B12 levels, which were okay), and a blood-pressure check.

Then I got down to the problem at hand. Leda wasn't eating regularly or well. Grieving the loss of her husband, she was mildly depressed. Because she was depressed, she didn't have much appetite. Because she didn't have much appetite, she wasn't cooking. "It doesn't make sense to heat up the kitchen when I'm only cooking for one," she said.

She needed to get her weight back up quickly, so I prescribed three things: a low-dose antidepressant, a daily half-hour walk to regain lost muscle tone and pique her appetite, and a regimen of calorie- and protein-dense meals. After our office visit, she and her daughter met with the dietitian to get ideas for creating calorie- and nutrient-dense meals.

At Leda's follow-up visit a month later, she'd regained a little over three pounds and said she'd stopped taking the antidepressant a couple of days before her visit. "I was a bit overwhelmed with my husband's death, but I'm coping better now and don't need it," she said.

Eating to live trumps living to eat

Some 2,400 years ago, Hippocrates, the father of Western medicine, said, "Let food be thy medicine and medicine thy food."

His words are as apt today as they were those thousands of years ago. What you eat (and how long you've been eating it) is the second most important factor in how well you're going to age (the first is exercise, which we'll be covering in the next chapter). Eat poorly, and your body doesn't develop the way it should; it's vulnerable to diseases and the complications that come along with them; it can't heal after illness or injury; it fails to flourish. Eat smart and, barring catastrophic accidents, it thrives.

Eating smart means eating foods that provide the following: calories for energy; compounds that fuel life processes such as hair growth, muscle contractions, brain function, ovulation, etc.; and the materials for building cells, tissues, muscles, organs, and bones. You really *are* what you eat.

Eating smart means eating defensively, both in terms of nutrition and weight. As you age, the lean muscle you depend on for strength and mobility declines, and so does your calorie requirement because this is the muscle that burns the most calories. At the same time, however, your need for foods that pack a lot of nutrition into a smaller number of calories increases. That's because your immune system needs more nutrients to fight the good fight. Your intestines aren't extracting and absorbing nutrients they way they used to (and that situation may become even worse if you're taking medicines that interfere with nutrient absorption), and your body's tissues and organs aren't using what's been absorbed and sent their way as efficiently as they used to either. (Note: Exercise, especially exercises that put a "load" on muscles and force them to increase their mass, can counteract lean muscle loss. We'll be talking about that in the next chapter.)

Eating smart means customizing your diet. There's no such thing as the one-size-fits-all diet. That's one of the main reasons that older people shouldn't get pulled in by fad diets – the grapefruit diet, the low-carb diet, the blood-type diet, etc. These diets – especially the grapefruit diet – can interfere with how medications are absorbed. And they can restrict the consumption of many of the nutrient-dense foods older people should be eating, which is what happens with the low-carb and blood-type diets. In addition, because many of these diet plans are created by people promoting how-to books, cookbooks, and prepackaged diet products, they can be expensive.

Eating smart means realizing that food is not the enemy. The enemy is misuse of food.

What's a Gram Worth?

When keeping track of your calorie intake, keep in mind the following:

Protein = four calories per gram

Carbohydrate (including sugars and starches) = four calories per gram

Fat = nine calories per gram

If you're severely underweight, a 350-calorie Krispy Kreme donut is a smart nutrition choice, but only for you in that situation. Without the energy and building materials all those calories provide, you can't think, you can't repair tissue, you can't go about your activities of daily living. But that would be a dumb nutrition choice for someone who's not malnourished.

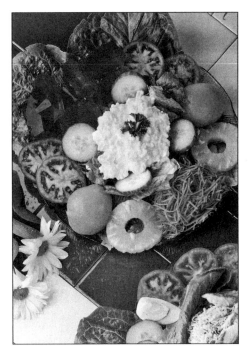

Eating smart means eating foods that are a finely calibrated mix of foods from the following *macro* (eat a lot) and *micro* (eat a little) food groups:

1. Carbohydrates

There are good carbohydrates and bad carbohydrates. The bad ones are simple sugars and highly refined starches that are digested quickly and go right into your bloodstream. The good ones are complex carbohydrates: whole grains, nuts and seeds, brightly colored vegetables, and deeply colored fruits. These are slowly digested and absorbed in the intestines. They provide not only energy but also most of the compounds (vitamins, minerals, and micronutrients such as phytochemicals, antioxidants, trace elements, etc.) the body needs to be strong and healthy, keep itself in good repair, and ward off chronic diseases such as diabetes, heart disease, and arthritis. According to the new USDA Dietary Guidelines, most of the foods you eat should come from this group.

2. Protein

We all need protein in our diet. However, unless you're fighting off an infection or recovering from an illness or injury (when you need between 100 and 120 grams of protein a day), like most people you could eat a third less protein each day and be perfectly healthy. The protein you do eat doesn't have to come in the form of steaks or chops either; beans and nuts, soy milk and tofu, fish and shellfish, low-fat dairy products, and eggs are all excellent sources of protein. In fact, eggs are near-perfect sources of protein.

3. Fat

Recommendations for a healthy diet say that 25 to 30 percent of total calorie intake should come from fats. Like carbs, there are good fats and bad ones. Bad fats are the "saturated," "trans," and hydrogenated fats found in hardened vegetable oils, margarine, and tropical oils. These fats encompass virtually all fried, fast, and packaged snack foods; "marbled" meat; and butter, cream, and other full-fat dairy products. They increase artery-clogging low-density lipoproteins (LDLs) and their even worse cousins V (for very) LDLs.

Good fats are the unsaturated or monounsaturated fats found in fish, "clear" oils (olive oil, canola oil, flax seed oil, etc.), nuts and seeds, and avocados. They help mop up the bad fats, they're required for the absorption of fat-soluble vitamins such as A, D, E, and K, and they're the building blocks for certain fats, such as heart-health-promoting omega 3, that the body can't make on its own. Making the switch from bad to good fats can lower your risk for a heart attack by more than 40 percent.

4. Fiber

Fiber (lignin, pectin, polysaccharides, etc.) is found in fruits, vegetables, nuts, grains, beans, and peas (complex carbohydrates). It comes in two forms: soluble, which turns to goo in the intestines, and insoluble, which doesn't. Both kinds of fiber keep food moving through the digestive tract, prevent constipation and diverticulitis (a very painful inflammation of tiny pouches lining the colon), and help reduce cholesterol. Both also help improve blood-sugar control and reduce the risks for diabetes and heart 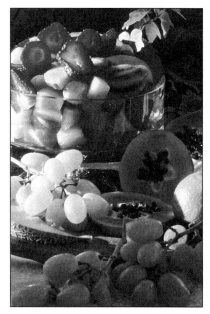 disease, and they may help prevent colon cancer. Scientists haven't yet figured out whether the indigestible fiber itself is responsible for all these benefits or whether they're due to the digestible micronutrients it contains. What is clear is that as you age, fiber becomes more and more necessary.

5. Micronutrients

Food was our first medicine, and that medicine was micronutrients: vitamins, minerals, trace elements (such as zinc and copper), antioxidants (such as the lycopene found in tomatoes or lutein found in eggs), phytochemicals (such as the flavonoids found in soy products and the tannins found in tea), and probiotics (such as *Lactobacillus acidophilus*, a gut-friendly bacterium found in yogurt). Due to the very sophisticated cell-signaling system human beings possess, the body's cells and tissues usually absorb this "natural medicine" in just the right amounts.

Iron is a good example. When you don't have enough iron in your diet, the lining of the duodenum (beginning portion of the small intestine) increases the formation of the receptors on the duodenum's interior walls so that more iron can be pulled out of the food passing through it. When you're taking in too much iron, however, the duodenum decreases the formation of those same receptors so that it's not overabsorbing iron.

6. Water

This is an often overlooked "nutrient." There's no hard-and-fast rule about how much water you should be drinking. Drink when you're thirsty, but keep in mind that the sense of thirst becomes dulled as you age *and* that you should be drinking enough liquid each day to prevent dehydration and constipation, and to maintain the body's sodium, potassium, and electrolyte balances. Older people need even more water during hot weather or when they have a fever or diarrhea. Juice and milk, clear and cream soups, soda (sugarless!), coffee, and tea can substitute for water, though the latter two are low on the substitute list since they often contain jitters-making caffeine and also act as diuretics.

To find out whether you're getting enough water, do a urine-bowel check. If urine is pale yellow and odorless, and stools are soft, you are; if urine is dark yellow or brownish and has an odor, and stools are hard, you aren't. Increase water intake accordingly.

One last word about eating smart, and this is something we have absolutely no control over: Our bodies prioritize which nutrients will be used first to provide energy. First come proteins, then carbohydrates, then fat. Just after a meal we tend to get our energy from protein and carbohydrates, while between meals we tend to get it from carbohydrates and fat. If we don't burn all the fat we consume, it's stored as fat tissue.

Plotting a course for healthy eating

So now that we know about the food groups, let's figure out the changes we should be making to ensure smart eating choices for life.

In 2005, the USDA released the new *Dietary Guidelines for Americans* and a totally revamped Food Guide Pyramid (replacing guidelines released in 1992). If you didn't know better, you'd think that the dietitians at the Department of Agriculture had done all the research for America's new diet plan in Asia or along the coast of the Mediterranean Sea. The heavily plant-based pyramid they came up with is strikingly similar to the "traditional" diets that have been keeping the people of Italy, southern France, Spain, Greece, China, and Japan mentally sharp, physically active, and heart-healthy well into their 80s.

The messages in the *Dietary Guidelines* (www.healthierus.gov/dietaryguide lines/) and Food Pyramid (www.mypyramid.gov) as well as from just about every dietitian and diet guru in the U.S. are simple:

- Eat a plant-based diet that's heavily weighted in favor of whole-grain breads and pastas; beans, legumes, and nuts; fresh, dried, canned, or frozen fruits; and dark-colored leafy vegetables.

- Eat nutrient-dense foods. How do you know whether a food is nutrient-dense? If it comes out of a shell or has a skin you can peel; if it's deeply colored (red, green, yellow, orange, pink); if it has a lot of pulp and fiber; and if it's raw, minimally processed, or unprocessed, it's probably nutrient-dense.

- Whether it's meat or dairy, eat it lean, low-fat, or fat-free.

- If you're over 50, get additional vitamin B12 (in its crystalline form), vitamin D, and possibly calcium. Take them in supplements or eat fortified foods.

- Limit your intake of bad fats (i.e., "trans" and saturated), refined sugar, salt, and alcohol.

■ To maintain your weight, balance your calorie intake with calories expended. In other words, if you don't want to gain weight as you age, match the number of calories you eat to the number of calories you need to maintain your specific activity level. To prevent gradual weight gain over time, you'll need to make small decreases in the food and beverage calories you consume, or increase your physical activity. (Doing both, as you'll see in Chapter 4, is the smart way to prevent weight gain.)

Tasty Tips for Boosting Nutrition

When older adults aren't eating as much as they should, the nutrient density of what they are eating needs to be augmented. These simple tips and tricks – often using store-bought or cooked-ahead ingredients – do more than just boost a meal's nutritional value and calorie count; they also increase flavor, texture, and mouth appeal.

TIP #1: BREAKFAST

■ Add sesame seeds or chopped fruit or nuts (apples, raisins, canned pineapple, walnuts, pecans) to cooked breakfast cereal, cottage cheese, or yogurt.

■ Add the pulp of a juiced orange to the water used to cook breakfast cereal.

■ Add powdered milk – full- or low-fat – to cooked or uncooked breakfast cereal.

■ Substitute whole-wheat bread or rolls for those made with refined flour.

■ Increase fiber content of canned juice by adding the juice (and pulp) of a fresh-squeezed lemon or orange.

Eating smart can be tough

For those in their 50s and 60s, eating smart usually means buying a couple of new cookbooks and turning bad eating habits into good ones.

It can be difficult for individuals who are older or have chronic conditions, because a number of factors besides just a bad diet contribute to poor nutrition. Probably the major factor is poor oral health. Not only have many people lost the teeth needed for chewing (molars), but they also may be dealing with ongoing tooth and gum infections, or periodontal diseases, which make chewing and swallowing painful. In extreme cases, the infections have led to the extraction of all teeth and the use of dentures. Mouths change, but dentures don't, and poorly fitting dentures often cause people to forsake meats and chewy foods, which provide nutrient-dense calories, for soft, gummy, and processed foods.

Salt: Too Much of a Good Thing

Most people consume far more sodium each day than they need or – given our high incidence of hypertension and stroke – than is good for them. One way to decrease salt in your diet is to use low-sodium products such as soups or snack foods; another way is to rinse canned and frozen vegetables in a colander before cooking or using them.

If a person has glossitis, an inflammation of the tongue, he can't taste his food, so he doesn't eat enough because it gives him no satisfaction. When that happens, the person tends to add more salt or sugar to what he is eating, or he'll turn to salty, processed foods. Neither change is for the good. Salt raises blood pressure, which already may be in the "iffy" range, and adding more sugar to foods adds empty calories and raises blood-sugar levels, which may lead to diabetes.

Poor oral health isn't the only cause of poor eating and malnutrition. When you're recovering from a stroke or have a condition like arthritis or emphysema that slows your eating, you tend to feel satiated before you get full. This may cause you to stop eating before you take in enough calories and nutrients to meet your body's calorie, energy, and health-maintenance needs.

Loss of smell is common among the elderly, especially among those who are taking ACE inhibitors and some other medications. If you can't smell, you don't enjoy eating, so you stop earlier than you normally would. Also, if you can't smell, you often don't recognize when food has spoiled, which can lead to diarrhea and dehydration.

In addition, consumption of certain fibers (such as the phytates in bran) and the use of certain medications, including prescription painkillers, affect digestion and how nutrients are or aren't absorbed. You can be eating the right things, but if the food is moving through the digestive tract so fast that nutrients can't be extracted from it, your nutrients simply end up in the toilet.

This is especially true for people who are chronic laxative users, as many older adults who suffer from constipation tend to be.

If people have poor vision or are living alone – especially men whose wives did all the cooking – the quality of their diet is likely to suffer. Nutrient-dense foods are often time-consuming to prepare: Beans take soaking and long hours of cooking, vegetables must be peeled and diced. And when you can't get around in the kitchen or don't know your way around it, you aren't going to spend time preparing food; you're going to spend it opening cans and popping frozen dinners into the oven. Not only are such products less nutritious and fiber-dense than home-prepared foods, but they also tend to be higher in sodium.

Older people also have lots of misperceptions about what they should be eating. We've already talked about how bad fad diets are. Add the low-fat diet to the list. Older adults are eliminating fat from their diets, yet for people in their 70s, a little fat is good: It provides padding if they fall and an extra store of energy if they happen to need it.

Tasty Tips for Boosting Nutrition
TIP #2: LUNCH/DINNER

- Add a teaspoon of olive oil or some other unsaturated, clear oil to canned soup or stew as it is cooking.
- As it's cooking, add store-bought frozen vegetables or home-cooked frozen whole grains (wheat couscous, brown rice, barley, etc.) to canned soup or stew.
- Purée canned vegetables, peas, or beans, and add them to soups and stews as they're cooking.
- Sprinkle ground seeds (flax, sesame, poppy) or nuts (peanuts, walnuts, cashews) into soups, on salads and vegetables, or over casseroles.
- Add ground seeds and nuts to sauces and fillings, and/or stir a tablespoon of nut butter into soup while it's cooking.
- Use low-fat/high-calcium yogurt in place of sour cream on baked potatoes and to "cream" spinach and carrots.
- Add store-bought soy protein powder to casseroles, thick soups, and milk-based drinks.

Poverty and history are factors, too. People who live on a limited income and who have to make a monthly decision whether to buy healthful food or medications to maintain their health, or who grew up not eating a lot of vegetables, fruits, or lean cuts of meat and fish, are probably not going to change their dietary habits.

All these factors can lead to a condition that we geriatricians call the anorexia of aging.

Red flags for malnutrition

Malnutrition doesn't mean you aren't getting enough calories. It means you aren't getting enough smart calories, protein, and essential nutrients from the food you are eating.

The easiest way to spot eating problems is a change in body weight. It might be good for a middle-aged person to go from 160 to 150, but for someone in his 70s a ten-pound drop in weight is not good; for someone in his 80s, it's a definite sign that he's at risk for malnutrition.

Another indicator is a change in personal appearance. If hair is unkempt, if an individual isn't as neat and clean as usual – or the home isn't – there are probably problems in other areas.

At the doctor's office, red flags will include a change in skin color due to anemia as well as changes in the eye's conjunctiva, the thin mucous membrane that lines the eyelids and the outer surface of the eyeball. Both are indications that "something" isn't right in the patient's diet.

But these are problems that are relatively easy to deal with or, better yet, prevent. You can increase both the calorie- and nutrient-density of foods people already are eating by switching to fortified foods (cereals, juices, breads) or by "fortifying" them yourself by adding powdered milk, frozen vegetables, or milled seeds to home-prepared cereals, soups, salads, or casseroles. (See Tasty Tips and Tricks for Boosting Nutrition, pages 31, 33, and 35.)

If fortifying foods at home isn't possible, or if all nutritional needs can't be met with food, then use supplements.

When someone requires immediate help due to a major illness or extreme malnutrition, use liquid supplements such as Boost or Ensure. These products have been carefully formulated to contain just the right amounts of calories and nutrients that individuals need to regain their weight and strength, and rebuild muscle and tissue. You could live your whole life on liquid supplements and be healthy – bored, but healthy.

Tasty Tips for Boosting Nutrition

TIP #3: SNACKS

■ Cut up fruits and vegetables into finger-sized slivers and keep them in a bowl of water in the refrigerator for easy snacking.

■ Create make-ahead yogurt parfaits by alternating layers of yogurt and chopped fruit, and keep them at the ready in the refrigerator.

■ Create blender "smoothies" using Knox gelatin, milk, yogurt, or cottage cheese and blender-friendly fruits, berries, and nuts.

You can get more ideas for creating tasty, nutrition-dense meals from:

Encyclopedia of Healing Foods, M. Murray, ND, J. Pizzorno, ND, and L. Pizzorno, LMT

One Bite at a Time: Nourishing Recipes for People with Cancer, Survivors, and Their Caregivers, by R. Katz, M. Tomassi, and M. Edelson

The Disease Prevention Cookbook, C. Schenider, RN, RD

The New American Plate Cookbook: Recipes for a Healthy Weight and a Healthy Life, American Heart Association

What Should I Eat: The Complete Guide to the New Food Pyramid, T. d'Elgin

---

Situations in which you'll need to use liquid supplements usually apply only to "outliers" (people who have not been eating well for a long time) or to those who have serious digestive-tract disorders or who are recovering from illness or major surgery.

For everyone else, real chew-and-swallow food is the best way to keep malnutrition at bay. However, there are a few exceptions.

Three excellent government studies, which catalogued food histories of older adults and measured what they actually ate against what they should have been eating, showed that although people 65 and older are generally eating well, they still aren't getting enough food-based calcium and vitamin D.

About fifteen minutes a day of exposure to sunlight would solve the vitamin D problem and more milk or bone-in fish added to the diet would solve the calcium problem, but it's obvious from the data that that's not happening. So to maintain bone health, people in their 60s, especially women, should be taking a calcium-vitamin D supplement.

Drugs That Can Cause Taste Dysfunction in the Elderly*

Category	Examples
Amebicides and anthelmintics	Metronidazole
Analgesic, anti-inflammatory, antipyretic, and antirheumatic drugs	Allopurinol, auranofin, colchicine, dexamethasone, gold, hydrocortisone, levamisole,D-penicillamine, phenylbutazone, salicylates
Anesthetics (local)	Benzocaine, lidocaine, procaine hydrochloride
Anticoagulants	Phenindione
Anticonvulsants	Carbamazepine, phenytoin
Antihistamines	Chlorpheniramine
Antihypertensives and diuretics	Acetazolamide, amiloride and its analogs, captopril, diazoxide, diltiazem, enalapril, ethacrynic acid, nifedipine
Antimicrobials	Amphotericin B, ampicillin, bleomycin, cefamandole, ethambutol, griseofulvin, lincomycin, metronidazole, sulfasalazine, tetracyclines
Antineoplastics and immunosuppressants	Azathioprine, bleomycin, carmustine, doxorubicin, 5-fluorouracil, methotrexate, vincristine
Antiparkinsonian drugs and muscle relaxants	Baclofen, chlormezanone, levodopa
Antithyroid drugs	Carbimazole, methimazole, methylthiouracil, propylthiouracil, thiouracil
Cholesterol-lowering drugs	Cholestyramine, clofibrate
Hypoglycemic drugs	Glipizide, phenformin, metformin
Oral hygiene components	Chlorhexidine gluconate (in mouth rinses), Na lauryl sulfate
Others	Etidronate, idoxuridine, iron dextran complex, vitamin D
Psychoactive drugs	Lithium, trifluoperazine
Sympathomimetic drugs	Amphetamines, amrinone
Vasodilators	Dipyridamole, nitroglycerin patch

*Duration of taste dysfunction ranges from hours to months and includes diminished (hypogeusia) and altered taste (dysgeusia).

The food-drug and drug-drug paradox

We need food to live, and as we get older, many of us also need medications to survive. In fact, 80 percent of people over 50 are taking some type of medicine. That includes everything from over-the-counter baby aspirin used to prevent heart attacks to prescription-only drugs taken to combat hypertension, osteoporosis, arthritis, or diabetes.

At 50, if you mix a medication with the wrong food or drink, you may have a food-drug reaction with minor side effects like gas or a bout of nausea. But as you age, your body is dealing with more chronic conditions, you may be taking more than one medication, and your digestive tract isn't handling things as well as it used to. Food-drug and drug-drug reactions can cause serious side effects, such as vomiting, diarrhea, delirium, falls that land you in the hospital, and worse.

Most medications are absorbed through the digestive tract. Some must be taken on an empty stomach so they can be absorbed better and more rapidly. For example, if bisphosphonates (Fosamax, Actonel, etc.) are being used to prevent or treat osteoporosis and they aren't taken on an empty stomach, their active ingredient binds with the food and liquid in the stomach and, rather than being absorbed, will be passed out of the body as very expensive waste.

Other medications may irritate the stomach. These should be taken with foods or just after you've eaten.

Certain foods can inhibit the action of a medication, not only reducing or canceling its effectiveness but also leading to unpleasant (gas, nausea) or painful (stomach cramps, vomiting) side effects. Among the worst offenders in this category are grapefruit, foods high in vitamin K, foods high in potassium, and alcohol.

To avoid food-drug and drug-drug interactions, know why you're taking a medication. Make sure to get written instructions on proper usage from your physician, pharmacist, or dietitian, and then follow them to the letter.

Also have your physician or pharmacist do a food-drug and drug-drug evaluation whenever you lose or gain more than a couple of pounds and every time you add or subtract an item from your medication regimen.

And finally, don't assume that just because a product is sold over the counter at the drugstore or is found in the supplements section at the health food store that you needn't treat it as you would a medication. If you take something for its perceived health benefit, you should treat it as if it were another medication and make sure that it doesn't interfere or interact with anything else that you're taking.

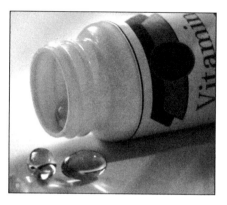

Chapter 4
Watching Your Weight

When Hugh M. retired at 66 from his job as head of security at a large office supply company in Cleveland, he weighed 161 pounds. He bragged at his retirement dinner that his job had kept him so busy that he was only nine pounds heavier than when he got out of the Army in 1973 and started with the company.

Retirement was not kind to Hugh. His weight went up seven pounds during his first year as a househusband and another eight the year after. But it wasn't the fifteen extra pounds that he packed on, mostly in his belly, that brought him in to see me; it was his shortness of breath. "I'm having problems keeping up with the guys when we go out hunting," he said. "Heck, I'm even getting winded when I climb the stairs at home, and that never used to happen."

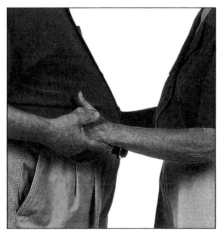

He wasn't just "getting winded." He was also experiencing what he called panic attacks at night. "I wake up gasping for breath, and sometimes I can't get back to sleep, so I'm a slug the next day."

In response to a few questions, Hugh admitted that his back was giving him problems, too, especially when he had to stand for any length of time.

"I know this is all related to my weight, doc," he said, "but it's only fifteen pounds. How bad could that be?"

An office physical that included a quick calculation of Hugh's body mass index (26.8), his waist-to-hip ratio (1.2), and a blood-pressure check showed him how bad.

In just two years, he'd added the equivalent of a fifteen-pound bowling ball's worth of fat to his body, and most of it was belly fat.

In terms of your health, that's a bad place to put on weight. Belly fat, or what physicians call intra-abdominal or visceral fat, causes your risk for certain kinds of cancers, diabetes, and heart disease to shoot up. Way up.

Belly fat is tough-to-lose fat. To take it off, you *must* cut calories and you *must* exercise.

Hugh's the kind of guy who responds to a challenge. He saw me on a Thursday, and on Friday he and his wife, Nora, went to the bookstore and bought the new *American Heart Association Cookbook*. The following Monday, he bought a membership at the local Y.

It took Hugh five months of low-fat eating (he admits he fell off the wagon a couple of times), treadmilling, curling, crunching, and working out with hand weights (to strengthen both back and abdominal muscles) to drop his post-retirement pounds and get rid of his belly.

He was on a roll, so he kept at it. "Just to see where things would go," he said.

The last time Hugh came in, he was a trim 156 pounds and was grinning from ear to ear. "You know what, Doc? Nora and I were cleaning out the guest-room closet, and I came across my Army uniform. Not only does it fit, it's actually a little big in the waist."

Life is full of weighty matters

We're going to be talking about weight, fat, and body mass for the next few chapters, so before you read any further, figure out where you stand weight-wise. Don't use life-insurance height-weight-age charts. Weight in the U.S. is skyrocketing, and the data from these charts give *average* weights, not *best* weights. To find out what your best weight is, you need to calculate your body mass index or BMI. (*See box on page 41.*)

A BMI of 18.5 or less means that you're underweight and probably somewhat malnourished. And if you're in your 70s or 80s, you're at increased risk for disability and an untimely death as well. A reading between 18.5 and 24.9 indicates a "healthy" weight: Men are "healthiest" between 22 and 24; women between 21 and 23. A reading between 25 and 29.9 means you're in the overweight zone. A reading of 30 or over means you're obese.

A BMI over 30 *plus* a waist measurement over 40 inches for men and over 35 inches for women is a double whammy, because it puts you at an even higher risk for the chronic conditions, illnesses, and diseases that come with obesity.

The BMI is a bowed-curve scale: Risks to both your short- and long-term health increase at the extreme ends of the curve. For those in their 50s and 60s, weight gain is the culprit; for people in their mid-70s and up, weight *loss* is.

Calculate Your Body Mass Index

Several Internet sites offer Body Mass Index calculators. The one at the Centers for Disease Control and Prevention is the one I use the most (http://www.cdc.gov/nccdphp/dnpa/bmi/calc-bmi.htm). The one at Partnership for Health Weight Management (www.consumer.gov/weightloss/bmi.htm) is good, too. The BMI calculator at www.halls.md/body-mass-index/bmi.htm lets you add gender and age to your calculation (and includes a weight percentile calculator).

If you don't have access to a computer, to calculate your BMI:

1. Multiply your weight in pounds by 703

2. Divide your answer by your height in inches

3. Again, divide your answer by your height in inches

4. The number you get is your BMI

Weight gain is a given

Weight creep generally starts for men in their 30s; for women, a decade later. By the time you hit 50, it's a given. If you don't take measures to stop gaining, it will bother you the rest of your life, which, due to the multiplier effect that both weight and fat have on other conditions, won't be as long or as full as you'd like.

The easy explanation for why you start gaining weight in your 30s and 40s is that you're taking in more caloric energy than you're expending in daily activities. It takes only 3,500 calories to produce a pound of fat, and if you take in 2,200 calories' worth of energy a day but only spend 2,100 to meet your daily energy needs, you're banking 100 calories a day in your fat account.

In 365 days you will have banked 36,500 *extra* calories. When you do the math (36,500 calories divided by 3,500 calories), that adds up to a weight gain of 10.4 pounds in a year. And that's just for one year!

But weight gain as you age is far more complicated than a mismatch between calorie input and energy use.

Why we gain weight

Skeletal muscle, the muscle wrapped around your bones that enables you to run, sit, and stand, is the body's main calorie burner, and it burns 24/7. Even if you're doing nothing, a pound of muscle will burn about forty calories in an hour (as opposed to a pound of fat, which burns only three calories an hour).

That's the good news. The bad news is that from your 30s on, your percentage of skeletal muscle tissue declines, while your percentage of muscle fat tissue increases. Even if you look and stay the same weight for decades, you become a well-marbled specimen on the inside.

Why the decrease in muscle mass and the increase in fat? With muscle, you either use it or lose it. You must stress and strain your skeletal muscle with activity and exercise for it to retain its calorie-burning efficiency. However, as you age you become less physically active. You're running PTA meetings rather than marathons, you're cutting the grass with a power mower rather than a push mower, you're shopping on eBay on Saturday morning rather than hitting the mall, and workouts at the gym . . . Well, you slip them in when you can.

When you aren't active, your muscle mass shrinks and you need fewer calories. Unfortunately, you don't realize that you've lost all that calorie-burning muscle, so you continue consuming the same number of calories, and *voilà*, middle-age spread. Left unchecked, it can continue into your 70s; the average weight gain per decade is five pounds for men and three and a half pounds for women.

Lost muscle mass isn't the only culprit

But loss of muscle mass and its replacement by fat are just two reasons for weight gain after you hit middle age.

Genes also play a major role, because they influence body type. Mesomorphic is a muscular build, ectomorphic a slender build, and endomorphic a soft build that's round or stocky. That means, by the way, that you can get a pretty good idea of what you might weigh as you get older by looking at your parents.

Genes also influence how efficiently your glands work. Case in point: your thyroid gland. Inheriting an overactive thyroid causes you to burn through calories quickly; inheriting an underactive one causes you to be prone to weight gain (until the condition is corrected with medication).

How Many Calories Do You Need?
Calculating your basal metabolism rate (BMR)

You need a certain number of calories just to maintain body functions such as breathing, body temperature, heartbeat, and blood circulation.

To find out how many calories your body needs just to exist, calculate your basal metabolism rate.

1. Divide your weight in pounds by 2.2 to get your weight in kilograms.
2. If you're female, multiply the result by .9 and use that figure for the next calculation; if you're a male, skip this step.
3. Multiply your weight in kilograms by 24.

This is the number of calories you'd need if you were simply sitting around and doing nothing, however – not when you're up and about and active. To have a life, you require 30 percent to 50 percent more calories. While there are extremely accurate (and expensive) tests that can tell exactly how many calories you should be eating to maintain weight, for a good ballpark estimate of how many calories you should consume each day, multiply your current weight by 10 if you're sedentary; by 15 if you're moderately active; and by 20 if you're extremely active or are recovering from an illness or injury.

Age-related changes in hormone secretion play a role, too. Declining levels of estrogen, testosterone, growth factors, and other gender-related compounds slow the body's ability to burn calories efficiently. Hormone decline also plays a role in where fat gets deposited. Normally, fat is deposited under the skin and in and around muscles, but for some people, when hormones decline, it starts accumulating around the waist and belly.

Apples and Pears

An increasing amount of research has shown that where you carry your fat has as much impact on your overall health status as how much fat you're carrying.

If your fat is concentrated just above and below your waist, giving you an apple-shaped appearance, or if it is concentrated in the abdomen, giving you a sway-backed appearance, it's far more hazardous to your health and well-being than if you're carrying it around your hips, which gives you a pear-shaped appearance.

People who carry their fat around their waist have a significantly higher risk for high levels of bad (LDL) cholesterol, hypertension, cardiovascular disease, diabetes, sleep apnea, cervical cancer, and breast cancer than those who carry it in their hips, buttocks, and thighs.

To find out whether you are (or are in danger of becoming) an "apple" or a "pear," get a measuring tape and use it to find your waist-to-hip ratio.

1. Measure your waist at its narrowest point (no sucking in your stomach!).
2. Measure your hips at their widest point (usually seven or eight inches below your belly button).
3. Divide your waist measurement by your hip measurement.

Men should have a waist-to-hip ratio of no more than .90; women's should be no more than .80.

Belly fat is extremely bad fat. (*See box above.*) Not only does belly fat throw your back out of whack and cause problems with walking, but it also secretes compounds that increase inflammation in your blood vessels. This raises your risk for dozens of debilitating, disabling, and life-shortening chronic diseases.

Age-related slowdown in metabolization of food is also a culprit. The longer food takes to travel through the digestive tract, the more slowly it is absorbed and burned, and the more it is stored as fat.

If their sense of smell and taste has declined (as is the case with smokers), many people reach for the salt shaker and the sugar bowl. Or they're bored and seek diversions in the kitchen. Both "solutions" cause weight gain.

Many medications, especially those used for asthma and depression, also cause weight gain.

Often, quitting smoking, although wonderful for your body in so many ways, also causes weight gain. An oral craving, the urge to put something in your mouth, is responsible for the weight gain. On average, men gain ten pounds after quitting and women gain eight.

It's not just about looks

Middle-age weight gain is more than just a dress-size or self-image problem. It's the open sesame to an array of often-interacting conditions and diseases that will have a negative impact on your health, your quality of life, and in many cases your bank account.

When you're younger, your body is hardy and resilient. You can get away with being overweight (and underweight, too) and not pay the piper. By the time you hit your 50s, however, you can't. You have two things working against you.

Your immune system, which is your body's natural defense system, is far less robust than it used to be. It now tends to go a little haywire if you put on weight. That's because it reacts to fat as if it were an injury or germ and sends out fighter cells (T-cells, etc.) to attack it. If fat were a germ, the fighter cells would do it in. But it's not, and this confuses the immune system, which then goes into attack mode with a systemwide inflammation (think of that as a low-grade fever) that puts constant physical stress on the body. That stress level gets ratcheted up when it interacts with whatever current health baggage you carry.

In your 50s, you're already loaded down with health baggage. This might include knee joints that are stressed and strained from decades of jogging, ulcers and high blood pressure from your job, lousy lungs from your spouse's two-pack-a-day habit, porous bones from a lifelong diet low in calcium and vitamin D, compressed spinal disks from sitting all day at your job, a semipickled liver from a twenty-year booze habit, etc.

Add weight gain to your baggage and you ratchet up your vulnerability to diseases that come with being overweight or that are more likely to occur *as you age* if you are overweight.

When I'm talking about being overweight, I'm not talking about being obese (i.e., having a BMI over 30 or weighing 20 percent or more than you should for your height and build). I'm talking about weighing twelve or eighteen or twenty-two pounds more than your BMI or your physician says you should.

Additional pounds put additional stress on your spine as well as your hip and knee joints. That tends to increase muscle and tendon injuries. And for people who are predisposed to arthritis, weight gain is often the straw that breaks the camel's back. The damage arthritis inflicts on joints and ligaments is irreversible.

Putting on additional pounds increases your risk for heart and circulatory problems: high blood pressure, angina and chest pain, heart attacks, and strokes. Additional pounds (especially if you're over 65) increase your risk for pre-diabetes (lowered insulin output accompanied by muscle-related insulin resistance) and full-blown diabetes. In fact, a weight gain of as little as eleven pounds – especially if you had gestational diabetes during a pregnancy – doubles your risk of developing type 2 diabetes. A greater weight gain ups the odds even more.

And of course, being overweight increases your risk for obesity.

Besides severely limiting your ability to lead a normal, active life, obesity increases the risk for all the above conditions and puts you at increased risk for asthma, pneumonia, chronic obstructive pulmonary disease (COPD), and a host of other respiratory conditions. It also puts a huge strain on your gall bladder and kidneys.

Being obese makes it difficult to sleep in any position except on your back. This doesn't just put a strain on your back; it also can cause sleep apnea, a condition in which belly fat compresses a person's lungs and windpipe, cutting off oxygen and causing the person to awake suddenly, gasping for air. People dealing with sleep apnea are actually dealing with two problems: oxygen starvation during the night and sleep deprivation and fatigue during the day.

Obesity puts you at risk for skin rashes, infections, and cuts and wounds that will not heal. It puts you at increased risk for skin cancer (the most common type of cancer); lung cancer (the number one cancer killer); and cancers of the colon, gall bladder, prostate, kidney, uterus and ovaries, and breast – with the latter occurring in men as well as women.

Few of these weight-related conditions work solo. It's rare, for instance, for diabetes and coronary artery disease or diabetes and kidney failure *not* to go hand in hand.

Underweight is as bad as overweight

You might assume that if too much weight is bad for your health, then too little is good. The opposite is true. People with BMIs in the range of 18.5 and under are usually carrying the same kind of health baggage as those in the 25-and-over range. The difference is that all that baggage is being carried around in a body that has *no* physical reserves available to protect the person from diseases and no reserves available for recovery when the diseases do strike. This is why people who are underweight die from such conditions as pneumonia and heart failure, which in people of normal weight would be merely a bad cold or heart palpitations.

Being underweight means that you're malnourished, which forces the body to break down what muscle you do have to get the energy and building materials, especially calcium and protein, that it needs to survive. This process increases the risk for osteoporosis, tooth loss, hip and joint problems, heart failure and stroke, kidney failure, muscle fatigue, falls, and disability.

Malnutrition is the single greatest cause of failure to thrive and often starts the downhill slide into total system shutdown seen in increasing numbers of people in their 80s.

It's often more difficult to treat the effects of long-term underweight than it is to treat those of long-term overweight, especially in the elderly. It's difficult to restore muscle lost to long-term protein starvation, and it's impossible to restore a hip bone shattered in a fall due to the osteoporosis caused by long-term calcium depletion.

All this means that watching your weight is the work of a lifetime and not just a life stage. If you want a healthy weight when you're 60, 70, and 80, and the independence and vitality that come with it, you have to watch what you eat. You have to front-load your bones with lots of calcium. You have to forgo the fat, salt, and sodium-rich foods and beverages that drive up blood pressure. You have to head into the physical decline of old age as nutritionally healthy and as high on the life arc as it's possible for you to be.

The return on all this vigilance is priceless. People who watch their weight as they age tend to have fewer illnesses and chronic diseases, and the ones they do get are usually easier to diagnose because the doctor isn't diagnosing them through a wall of fat. And they're easier to treat, too, because the physician doesn't have to adjust treatment to take into account the effect the patient's fat and weight will have on medications, treatments, or therapies.

And when you're dealing with fewer health and medical conditions, you're going to have a better quality of life. You'll get out more, be more social, participate in more activities, and be more independent. Your glass will be half full, not half empty.

Watching what you eat – really

It's a given: By the time you hit your late 50s, your body isn't burning calories as well as it used to, *and* any post-midlife pounds you put on are probably already having a negative impact on your health. That means you want to keep post-midlife weight gain at bay (at least until you reach your late 70s or early 80s, when a little fat is good for you).

To do that, you have lots of options.

Rethink your diet

- Eat for mouth appeal. Crunchy, chewy, textured foods engage you in the act of eating. When those foods are fiber-dense fruits, nuts, vegetables, beans, and/or whole grains, they also occupy more space in your stomach, which leaves less room for high-fat, high-calorie foods.

- Eat for high nutrient density. Boost your intake of high-quality protein, such as fish, lean meats, dairy products, and eggs; calcium and vitamin D; vitamin-, mineral-, and micronutrient-rich fruits and vegetables; and fiber-dense carbohydrates. Make sure to budget time into your life for the extra shopping and preparation these health-boosting foods require.

- Read labels when you shop for and prepare foods, and pay particular attention to fat grams and calories. When 50 percent or more of a product's calories are from fat, it's not a smart or healthy choice.

- Cut down or completely eliminate empty-calorie foods. White sugar, foods made with fructose and other syrup sugars (corn syrup), and foods made with refined grains and processed fats and oils (hydrogenated, saturated, etc.) are at the top of the list. Running a close second are full-fat foods, for which there are always lean or low-fat substitutes.

■ Switch to diet soft drinks. Regular soft drinks are loaded with empty-calorie syrup sugars.

Change how you eat

■ Never let yourself get to the point that you're famished, because that leads to overeating.

■ Eat more slowly. It takes the brain about twenty minutes for the "I'm full" feeling to kick in. The more slowly you eat, the fewer calories you'll consume before the feeling of fullness kicks in. Try chewing each bite thoroughly, putting your fork down between bites, or engaging in conversation.

■ Make lunch your big meal. The Europeans have been doing this for ages, and look at the shape they're in.

■ Reduce portion sizes. An easy way to do this is to change the size of your dinner plate. Instead of using the standard 13-inch plate, eat your meals from a 9-inch plate. Research has shown that what you think you're eating (i.e., a plateful of food) has as much to do with how full you feel at meal's end as with what you actually chew and swallow.

■ Spread things out. Don't eat three squares a day; make it four or five. Not only does this help you feel full all day, it also ensures a constant flow of energy to your brain and muscles so that you don't have those energy lows during the day.

■ Avoid late meals. Eating and then going right to bed can lead to gastroesophageal reflux disorder. In addition, it just about ensures that everything you eat will be turned to fat, because you're headed into sleep mode, the lowest calorie-burning mode of all.

Just watching your weight won't cut it

Carefully monitoring your food intake by weighing and measuring it and counting the calories in every morsel you eat is one way to drop and maintain weight. If you go on a strict low-calorie or low-fat or low-carbohydrate or low-whatever diet (with which you'd need to take supplements, since limiting food intake also limits your intake of vitamins, minerals, and fiber), you do lose weight. But you're shooting yourself in the foot. Not only does this kind of weight-watching take all the fun out of eating and leave you hungry all the time, but it's also not a long-term fix. Part of the weight you lose is calorie-burning muscle, and with less muscle available to burn calories, you're soon back in the same boat, taking in more calories than you have muscle to burn them. That's why 95 percent of people who lose weight through dieting regain what they lost and then some within five years.

It's easier (and more nutritionally sound!) to watch your weight with a combination of diet modification and exercise. Exercise doesn't just burn calories; it increases muscle mass, which increases your ability to burn more calories (and increase your nutrient intake in the process), which builds more muscle mass, which … well, you get the picture.

In addition, exercise revs up your heart, circulatory system, and lungs, and pumps up your brain's production of the feel-good hormones (endorphins, serotonin, adrenalin) that boost mood and make you feel more refreshed and energized.

In my opinion, exercise is the next best thing to the fountain of youth. And it's a self-fueling engine for staying young, active, and vital. The more you do, the more you can do.

Chapter 5
Pumping Iron for Health, Vigor, and Long Life

Maxine F. is the kind of patient every doctor loves. At 79, she's sharp as a tack. A former teacher whose husband, Ted, died six years ago, she lives alone and cherishes her independence. She loves to read, and in fact I can always count on her to bring me an interesting tidbit of information when she comes for an office visit.

When she showed up in my office this spring almost in tears, I knew something was wrong.

"I have no energy," she said. "A trip to the grocery store leaves me so exhausted that when I get home, I have to sit down to catch my breath because I'm scared I'll fall if I try to put the groceries away. And last week, when I baked a pie and I was taking it out of the oven, the weight of the pie was too much for me. I dropped it.

"This never used to happen," she sighed. "What's wrong with me?"

I reevaluated her medications (she takes a diuretic for hypertension, nitrate for a heart condition, and Fosamax for osteoporosis) and they were fine. Her blood pressure was a little high, but that often happens when people have it taken at their doctor's office. Her blood panel and urine test, which she'd had done at the lab two days before her office visit, showed that everything was in the normal range.

It was during her physical exam that the cause of Maxine's fatigue and muscle weakness became clear.

She'd lost three pounds since her last visit. When people her age lose weight, they usually don't lose fat, they lose muscle mass. When I asked whether she had increased her activity level and was burning more calories, she laughed. "No. I'm worried about falling or having an accident driving, so I've cut down on a lot of things. I'm conserving my energy."

Conserving energy was Maxine's problem. Loss of muscle and strength is part of an insidious cycle of "use it or lose it." While she was conserving her energy, she'd been weakening and losing muscle.

At the end of Maxine's office visit I wrote two prescriptions. One was for a three-month regimen of liquid nutritional supplements to help her regain the weight she'd lost *and* provide the energy and building materials for the muscle she needed to regain and strengthen. The other was for strength training and gait training with our rehabilitation-therapy department.

Twice a week for the next ten weeks, Maxine huffed and puffed and sweated. She did leg lifts with and without ankle weights to recondition her thigh muscles (quadriceps). She worked out her arms and legs with increasingly resistive Therabands. She underwent balance training with simple t'ai chi movements such as slow backward-and-forward lunges and ten-second leg stands. Finally, she worked out – after some cajoling from the therapist – on a balance board that was set low to the floor. The first two exercises increased her leg and upper-body muscle bulk and strength; improved her overall posture, knee-joint function, and upper-body reach (range of motion); and helped improve her balance when standing. The other two exercises improved her balance when standing and walking, her step length (stride), and her walking speed (gait).

During her last week of therapy, at Maxine's suggestion, the therapist did a session at Maxine's home. "I wanted her to see where I lived so she could maybe offer suggestions on things I might need to change or improve at home, and I wanted her to see my 'home gym,' too," said Maxine.

Today, Maxine works out at home two or three times a week, and she has regained much of the mobility and vigor she had two years ago. But the operative word here is "much."

Maxine reconditioned her muscles and in the process improved her cardiopulmonary function, but she'll never get back to where she was before she became deconditioned.

The sad part of this story is that her loss of conditioning was preventable. If she'd been participating in a regular exercise program she'd never have gotten deconditioned in the first place.

Spread the good news

As I said in the last chapter, the closest thing there is to a fountain of youth is exercise. It's obvious when you look at older people who have always worked

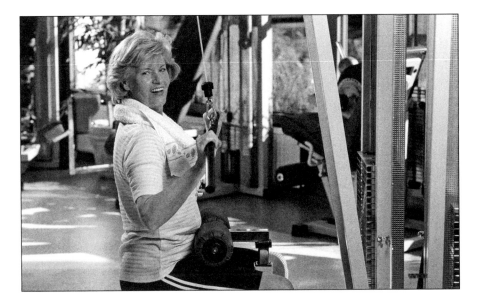

out (my personal hero is Jack LaLanne, who's in his 90s) that exercise keeps you looking and feeling younger.

But looks are just the tip of the iceberg. There is abundant scientific evidence that exercise also improves physical function and health status.

That's the good news. The better news is that exercise is an equal-opportunity life-enhancer. Whether you are a 45-year-old who hasn't put on gym shoes since high school or, like 79-year-old Maxine, never went into a gym in your life, it's never to late to start or resume exercising. And, whether you want to improve muscle strength and tone, increase stamina and vigor, work off weight, boost athletic performance, or improve balance and gait, a regimen or program is out there that will fit your needs.

Advanced age is never a reason for not exercising. One study, done with a group of frail nursing-home residents in their 80s and 90s, showed that an exercise program begun late in life offers benefits – improved cardiovascular function, increased mobility, etc. – that have a dramatic effect on health, independence, and quality of life. All the people who participated in the ten-week weightlifting and strength-training program increased their muscle mass and walking speed. Several walked up stairs for the first time in years, and others were able to stop using their canes and walkers!

The best news is that as little as thirty minutes a day of moderate activity such as raking leaves, vacuuming, or water-walking is all it takes for the health-boosting benefits of exercise to kick in. If you increase the time you spend exercising and/or ratchet up the intensity level a couple of notches, you'll see even better results.

And because exercise offers both preventive and therapeutic benefits, whether you're looking at the uphill or downhill side of aging, a well-planned exercise program covers just about all your health bases.

Exercise may retard the aging process

All too often, middle-aged people drift into a sedentary lifestyle, which, unchecked, continues into old age. The overall loss of conditioning that accompanies this process results in muscle and skeletal changes extremely similar to the muscle and skeletal changes that come with aging. This similarity has generated dozens of studies and led researchers to conclude that many of the signs, symptoms, and effects of aging can be put off, modified, or *reversed* with exercise. (In fact, Dr. Michael Roizen, a colleague of mine and author of *The Real Age Makeover*, devotes a whole chapter in his book to the age-reversing benefits of exercise.)

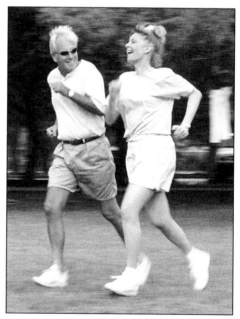

Exercise doesn't magically roll back the clock. However, it does improve the overall functioning of the immune system by reducing physical stress, and it increases the production of the fighter cells that seek out and destroy invading microbes, viruses, and diseased cells. Exercise also reconditions organs, muscles, tissues, and joints that have become weak and out of shape from disuse.

The fact that all these body parts have to be reconditioned is one of the main reasons that, whether you're starting an exercise program in your fit 40s or your frail 80s, you need to get a full medical evaluation: blood-pressure check, screening for heart and lung capacity, diabetes test, exercise stress test, etc. It's also the reason you need to discuss with your doctor (and, if you have joint problems, maybe your orthopedist) the types of exercise you want to start doing.

The discussion should cover:

■ Short-term and long-terms results you're hoping for versus the ones you're likely to get

■ Adaptations or modifications you could or should make to a workout or exercise program to ensure your safety and well-being

■ The best way to get started and to pace and monitor your progress

---

Strategies for Safe Workouts

Start slowly and increase the frequency, duration, and intensity of exercise activities gradually.

■ Breathe properly, and be sure not to hold your breath.

■ Always monitor your heartbeat rate. If you're taking blood-pressure medications, don't use your pulse or throat heartbeat to judge how intensely you're exercising.

■ Use the proper equipment (especially shoes) for exercise and athletic activities.

■ Stay hydrated: Drink before, during, and after a workout (unless your physician has told you not to).

■ Never begin a workout without first "warming up" your muscles by rubbing them briskly. Never end a workout without doing a series of flexes, extensions, and stretches.

■ When bending forward or backward, bend from the hips, not the waist.

■ If any position, bend, stretch, or activity hurts, stop doing it immediately.

■ If you don't know how to use a piece of equipment correctly, don't use it.

■ If you can carry on a normal conversation while you're performing an exercise activity, it's too easy. If you can't talk at all, it's too hard. Aim for somewhere in the middle.

People over 75, those with severe physical impairments, and those who have been physically inactive for several months or more should also discuss their fitness goals and exercise aspirations with a physical therapist, occupational therapist, exercise physiologist, strength-and-conditioning coach, or personal trainer. All will be able to supply information on alternative exercises and adaptive equipment, and explain how to balance exercise goals with energy expenditures (for those who are overweight) and conservation (for those who are underweight).

Springing into an exercise program will have the same effect on your body as gunning your car out of the garage after it's been sitting for a year. You'll go maybe a block and then poop out because all your lines are clogged with sludge. Or, worse yet, you'll blow your engine.

Once you get going, however, exercise is a self-fueling engine. The more you do, the more you can do, and the better and the longer you can do it, too.

Exercise and debilitating diseases

Exercise has been shown to have a preventive or modifying effect on many of the chronic illnesses and diseases, such as heart disease, diabetes, arthritis, and cancer, that cause disability and death. This is important to know because in so many of the cases that I see, the diseases are the bullets, but it's inactivity that's pulling the trigger.

As a *primary prevention*, an aerobic exercise program that works large muscle groups and promotes cardiopulmonary (heart-lung) and cardiovascular (heart-circulatory system) fitness significantly lowers your risk of heart attack. In addition, it increases lung capacity and muscle mass, which increases how efficiently calories are burned. Because this kind of exercise tends to keep body fat in check (and a high ratio of fat-to-muscle is a risk factor for *all* types of cancers), it looks as if it reduces the risk for breast cancer, too. In those who are older, gentle aerobic exercise improves flexibility and balance, which lowers the risk of falls.

As *secondary prevention*, exercise can treat current disease symptoms that could escalate into or contribute to a more serious health problem. For instance, a weight-bearing exercise program (called resistance training by rehabilitation therapists) doesn't just build and strengthen muscle and lower the risk of bone loss. For those with type 2 diabetes, it can improve both the amount of muscle available to respond to insulin and the way the muscle responds to it. That means that many diabetics who are in weight-bearing exercise programs are able to decrease their use of injected insulin or their oral medications.

As *tertiary prevention*, exercise can be used either alone or in conjunction with other therapies or medications to reduce symptoms and complications of recurrent diseases. For instance, someone suffering the unremitting pain and joint stiffness of osteoarthritis of the knee will decrease pain *and* have better range-of-motion improvement if therapy includes a combination of stretching-and-toning flexibility exercises for the upper thighs along with corticosteroid injections.

Indirect effects of exercise

Exercise doesn't have a positive effect on just muscles and bones and tissue. It also works its sweaty magic on the brain and psyche.

Dozens of studies have shown that because it revs up circulation and sends more oxygen to the brain, exercise helps improve focus, concentration, and creativity. And no matter what your age, it also helps you sleep better at night, operate under less whole-body stress (i.e., have less muscle tension, lower blood pressure, and a higher red-blood-cell count), and have fewer mood swings and less anxiety and depression. These benefits are due to the relaxing effect exercise has on muscles and to the stimulation and production of "feel-good" chemicals (endorphins, adrenalin, etc.) in the brain.

A recent study, published in *Annals of Internal Medicine*, found that exercise may also lower risk for Alzheimer's disease. The study found that people 65 an older who engaged in exercise three or more times a week had a 30 percent to 30 percent lower risk for *all* forms of dementia.

And of course, there's the undisputed weight-loss payoff of exercise. Only two things take weight off faster than exercising: stomach-bypass surgery and a structured (you might as well call it a starvation) diet. Neither offers the huge array of health benefits unrelated to weight that come with exercise, and research indicates that weight lost through those two methods is harder to keep off than weight lost through exercise.

Exercise builds muscle, and muscle burns fat!

Three workouts, one outcome: A better you!

To get all the benefits that come with exercise, no matter where you are on life's arc, you need to "bulk up." In non-Mr. Universe terms, that means you need to build and strengthen your muscle mass with weight-bearing exercises, aerobic exercises, and flexibility exercises. Each type of exercise produces the same effect: better muscle. They just take a different approach doing it.

Weight-bearing exercise

This is also known as resistance exercise and strength training, because when you engage in weight-bearing exercise, you're strengthening and building muscle by working it against some kind of resistance. Whether you're on the treadmill, doing the crawl in the pool, or doing wall push-offs, the resistance you're working against is gravity. When you're working out on resistance machines or with barbells, sand-filled ankle weights, or plastic milk cartons filled with water, the resistance comes from the weights.

Weight-bearing exercise puts stress on muscles, tendons, and joints, hence the tenderness, swelling, and pain that come – at least initially – with a muscle-building workout. But stress is a good thing for muscle. If you don't stress muscle (e.g., you're bed-bound by illness or sit in a comfy chair in front of the TV all day), you lose it. (*See Building Muscle Means Stressing Muscle, page 59*).

Stressing muscle with an every-other-day session of moderately intense weightlifting, band-stretching, or power-walking helps *maintain* muscle mass and strength. Ratcheting up the intensity with heavier weights, a stronger band, and/or a longer walk *builds* muscle and increases strength.

In addition to building and maintaining muscle, weight-bearing exercises also contribute to improved carbohydrate and blood fat (lipid) breakdown and use, and stimulate bone growth and strength. Strong muscles and strong bones mean less chance of osteoporosis, good balance and gait, and fewer falls that can land you in a hospital or nursing home.

There are two *big* don'ts when you're doing weight-bearing exercises. Don't exercise to exhaustion. That just leads to muscle fatigue, nervous-system fatigue, and dehydration – all of which contribute to accidents and falls. And don't stress your joints excessively. Just because your deltoid (shoulder) muscle can handle "pumping" a 25-pound weight doesn't mean that your rotator cuff (shoulder joint) can.

Building Muscle Means Stressing Muscle

Compare a muscle to a length of rope. You can stretch rope by pulling on it with a weight. You can bunch it up by squeezing it or unravel it by twisting it. You can cause it to fray by bending its fibers back and forth. The more you use a rope, the more you weaken it.

Muscle, on the other hand, is very active living tissue. So when it's pulled, squeezed, twisted, and worked back and forth, its reaction is to fight back. This causes microscopic rips and tears (which are the reason for the heat, pain, and swelling that often accompany a muscle-building workout) to occur. For the most part – in other words, when you haven't gone overboard with a workout – the rips and tears are nothing you need to worry about, but they are some-thing your body finds worrisome. So it sends out enzymes (think of them as a repair crew) that break down body fat and other compounds into repair materials and sends them to the rips and tears. As the rips and tears heal (which takes two or three days), they cause the muscle surrounding them to increase in size and therefore strength.

Because muscle is active living tissue, this rip-tear-repair cycle is an ongoing process, one that can always be increased and improved upon by participation in a structured exercise program that includes at least two days a week of muscle-building and strength-training. If you can't handle a full-body workout session, split things up. Do the upper-body workout on Tuesdays and Thursdays, and the lower-body workout on Mondays and Wednesdays.

Aerobic exercise

This is sometimes called cardiovascular or cardiopulmonary conditioning, because its primary purpose is to strengthen and condition the heart and lungs as well as the veins and arteries that supply them with blood, oxygen, and nutrients. Aerobic exercise does that by giving your body's large muscle groups, especially those in your legs and arms, a continuous rhythmic workout. This is *the* exercise for burning calories.

To be effective, an aerobic workout should last at least twenty minutes and be intense enough for you to reach your target heartbeat rate by the time you're done. To calculate your target rate, subtract your age from 220. For a moderately intense workout, your "target" heart rate should be 50 percent to

70 percent of that number; for an intense workout, it should be 60 percent to 90 percent. However, those calculations don't apply for individuals who are taking beta blockers or using pacemakers.

Flexibility exercise

This is sometimes called stretching-and-toning exercise. The aim of these bending, twisting, flexing, stretching, and curling exercises is to make your muscles work more fluidly. Because flexibility exercises gently pull, tug, and stretch muscles, tendons, and bones into alignment, they improve posture, reach, range of motion, balance, and gait. In addition, they reduce the stiffness in muscles and joints that comes with aging and a sedentary lifestyle. Flexibility workouts use the smooth, flowing movements of things like yoga, t'ai chi, and water aerobics, so they should never cause pain. And, research shows, they produce the same range of motion improvement in people in their 80s as they do for people in their 20s.

It's definitely never too late to start this gentlest form of exercise.

To get all the physical and psychological benefits that come with exercise, you should be doing all three types of exercise. And in most situations, because they tend to overlap, you are. It's impossible to do a good aerobic workout without putting muscle-building stress on the large muscles of your arms and legs and reducing muscle and joint stiffness. Conversely, it's impossible to do a good weight-bearing exercise session without pushing up your heart rate, giving your lungs a good workout, and flexing, stretching, and juicing up your joints.

Getting FITT

What you may not be doing (especially if you're attending a once- or twice-weekly workout session, have cobbled together your own program, or are using a videotape workout) is getting all the FITTness from exercise that you can. That's FITTness as in Fitness, Intensity, and Time on Task, all measures of your exercise progress.

You can't just do the same exercises and routines over and over again. You have to gradually:

■ Increase their frequency. For example, if you're pumping 10-pound barbells twice a week to build upper-arm muscle mass and strength, increase that to five times in two weeks. Or, if you're using 5-pound ankle weights to build upper-thigh strength, increase the number of lifts in your routine by two, then three, then four. Never work out the same muscles two days in a row, however. You have to give muscle time to repair itself from the small rips and tears that occur during a workout.

■ Increase your intensity. Once you reach the point where you barely notice that you're pumping a 10-pound barbell or 5-pound ankle weight, switch to heavier weights. Then, by increasing your frequency, work your way up to the point where those weights, too, barely cause a jump in your heart rate.

There are several ways to measure intensity. One is by monitoring your heart rate. Another is the Borg Scale, a simplified scale that rates exercise effort from nothing to very difficult. But the easiest one to use is the talk test: If you can carry on a conversation with no problem, your workout is not intense enough to be doing you much good. If you're breathless – can't utter more than two or three words at a time – it's too intense.

You should always monitor the intensity of your workout closely, especially if you have heart problems or are in an exercise program to improve cardiac function. Before you increase intensity, go back to your physician and get reevaluated.

■ Increase your time on task. When you increase the frequency and intensity of an exercise activity, you usually increase its duration, or time on task, as well.

Exercise physiologists call getting FITT "progressing." Trying to progress in all three areas at once, however, is a prescription for physical exhaustion and accidents.

Choosing a workout program that works for you

Whether you're 40, 60, or 80, deciding to get as fit as you possibly can means committing yourself physically and psychologically to what is probably going to be a major lifestyle change. It's a change that includes more activity, more self-monitoring, and more work for you. While getting fit has no downside, few people have the self-discipline to stick with this kind of makeover program unless they take ownership of it.

How Exercise Can Improve Chronic Conditions

Dozens of studies have shown that exercise helps you ward off or stay on top of many diseases and conditions, and that the health-promoting effect of exercise can kick in with as little as thirty minutes a day of activity.

The following list just scratches the surface:

Alzheimer's disease – Less cognitive decline, especially in women.

Anxiety – Lessens symptoms.

Atherosclerosis – Increases clearance (luminal diameter) of arteries leading to and from the heart.

Cardiovascular disease – Lowers risk of death after heart attack and improves artery function by keeping arteries swept clean of artery-clogging compounds (plaque).

Cerebrovascular disease – Reduces risk of stroke, especially in women.

Chronic obstructive pulmonary disease (COPD) – Improves lung function, capacity, and breathing.

Depression – Lessens symptoms.

Diabetes (type 2) – Increases muscle's sensitivity (uptake) to insulin and improves glucose tolerance.

For that to happen, the exercises and the program they create have to be individualized. One person with arthritis may love the smooth and gentle flexibility workouts offered in a t'ai chi class. Another person, seeking the same relief for her arthritic knees, will find it with a Pilates video. Yet another person will find what he wants in a yoga class.

The approach you choose must take advantage of your current skill level, abilities, and aspirations. For some people, the perfect exercise program is a forty-five minute walk around the local mall every morning with friends; when they want to kick up the intensity of the workout, they carry hand weights. For others, the perfect program includes three nights a week of aerobic kick-boxing at the local kung-fu center, two nights a week of weightlifting at the local body-building gym, and one night a week of flexibility training at home with a personal trainer.

Hypertension – Reduces resting blood pressure.

Low back pain – Strengthens abdominal muscles; promotes loss of abdominal fat; improves performance of daily activities.

Obesity – Reduces total body fat; reduces strain on cardiovascular system and back; reduces risk for type 2 diabetes.

Osteopenia/osteoporosis – Delays decrease in bone density; improves calcium absorption by bone.

Peripheral vascular disease – Increases muscle strength and stamina so more oxygen is circulated in the blood and delivered to arteries.

Physical frailty – Postpones muscle decline and disability; improves appetite.

Sarcopenia – Builds muscle size and strength; improves function and mobility.

Sleep apnea – Reduces abdominal fat; takes pressure off lungs and windpipe during sleep.

Surgery, protracted illness, trauma – Decreases risk for death and rehospitalization; improves quality of life and physical function, and counters depression.

Vascular disease – Increases the volume of oxygenated blood circulating in the body; lowers resting and exercising heart rates.

An exercise program may just be your prescription for better health!

It has to be a program you can work into your daily schedule. That's not to say that it has to be easy to work in, but it has to be *work-in-able*. If it's not, you're doomed to failure. Either you'll give up, or you'll end up rushing through things so quickly that you hurt yourself or get no fitness benefit from what you're doing.

The program has to have enough variety – in terms of either what you're doing or with whom you're doing it – to keep you motivated. Lack of variety and absence of motivation are the two main reasons so many people stop working out when they use videos. Not only do videos not push you to increase your fitness level, they become boring from repetition.

The program has to show results, and it has to show them fairly quickly. Results are hard to quantify. For some people, results mean dropping a certain number of pounds or inches in a month. Others see results in a drop of five beats per minute in their heart rate. For still others, it's how juiced their joints feel after a session of water aerobics, or perhaps it's the people they've met bobbing around next to them in the pool.

Most important of all, a fitness program that you end up sticking with has to have a goal to help crystallize your resolve. And goals aren't always rational or even health-related.

For some, the goal is amorphously lofty: To do whatever it takes to get as healthy and as physically fit as they can, and to stay that way for as long as possible.

For others, the goal is functional: To stave off a heart attack, control cholesterol, and bring down blood pressure so they don't die of a heart attack at 63 the way their fathers did; to sweat off the thirty-five pounds they put on after they gave up smoking ten years ago – and keep it off; to participate in this year's marathon; to improve balance and gait lost after knee-replacement surgery; or to to stay flexible and limber enough to continue competing in ballroom-dancing contests.

For some, it's vanity: To drop the thirty pounds they gained since they graduated from high school and show up at the next class reunion as sleek and svelte as their former high-school selves; to increase their metabolic rate to that of a shrew so they can eat anything; to enter the Mr. Senior Universe Contest – and win!

The bottom line on exercise is that it's the cheapest, safest, and best health insurance you can take out. Just do it!

Chapter 6
Gray Matters: The Aging Brain and Nervous System

I'd been seeing 77-year-old Leonard C., who has congestive heart failure and arthritis, for several years. The last time he came in for a checkup he seemed a bit distracted. He was polite and forthcoming, as always, but distracted.

So I wasn't totally surprised when his daughter, in town for a weekend visit with her dad, called and asked if I could see him the next week. "Something's wrong," she explained on the phone. "I've never seen the house so, well, messy – not even when Mom died and he went all to pieces. All he's done since I came yesterday is sit in the living room with a book in his lap. Or he complains: This hurts, that hurts, he's tired. But when I try to get him to talk, he gets angry, or worse, he tells me it doesn't matter, he's old, and he's got an old man's problems."

When Len came in on Monday, he was using a cane. "I'm here because Lois hounded me to come. I'm fine," he said gruffly.

And physically he was. He'd lost a couple of pounds since his last visit, but his blood pressure was okay, his vision was good, and despite the cane ("I tripped in the house"), his bones and joints were, too.

"Your daughter's worried, Len. Should she be?" I asked.

That took all the wind out of Len's sails. He looked at me and sighed. "I'm losing it. I'm forgetting things. I'm dropping things. I'm up half the night. Sometimes the TV's on, sometimes not. And I'm constipated."

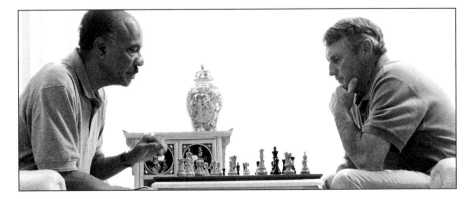

I asked Len whether he'd mind taking the Mini-Mental State Examination, a short, in-office mental-status test. Five minutes later, we were done. For his age and health status, he'd sailed through the test.

Cognitively, Len was fine. However, in light of the symptoms he was exhibiting, I wasn't so sure about his emotional state. "What's going on in your life, Len?" I asked.

"Oh, the same old same old," he replied with a shrug. Then he heaved another sigh and leaned forward in his chair. "Pete died three months ago," he said with a catch in his throat. "We were going bowling. He didn't answer the door. I had to get a neighbor to climb in a window and open the door for me. He was upstairs. It was a heart attack. He was just lying there on the floor."

Len was grieving the loss of a good friend, and his grief had turned into depression.

If this were a mild depression or had been caught earlier, I'd have prescribed a low-dose antidepressant. But it wasn't mild and it had taken root, so I prescribed an antidepressant and psychological counseling as well. And I made an appointment to see him again in six weeks, so we could both monitor their effect.

Len's recovery was slow. He was able to discontinue therapy after two months, but he continued taking antidepressants for a year. Eventually, he did recover the zest for life he'd lost with Pete's passing.

Still, I'm going to keep an eye on Len. He did well on the mental-status exam, but the profound depression he experienced is often a warning sign for dementia.

Brain Anatomy 101

The brain is your body's most complicated organ. But just for now, think of it as a multilayered Tootsie Pop.

Your skull is the hard outer shell. Inside that is your wrinkled and convoluted cerebral cortex (containing both gray and white matter), where most of your thinking, reasoning, learning, knowledge-storing, decision-making, and "aha!" moments take place. This mass of tissue consists of billions of brain cells (neurons) made of protein, carbohydrates, and fat. These cells are packed together so densely that they create a solid-looking mass. Each cell has a nucleus surrounded by dendrites that look like tiny tree branches and a long axon, or conduit, sheathed in fat. Axons carry the nerve impulses that allow the cells to communicate with each other and other parts of the brain. They do this ceaselessly, in bursts of chemicals (mostly the neurotransmitters acetylcholine, serotonin,

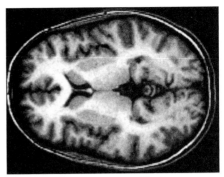

Brain scan showing cortex and brain stem.

and norepinephrine) kicked up and down the axon by an electrical charge.

The cerebral cortex, which gets thinner and thinner as you age, is wrapped snugly around the midbrain. This is the site of your olfactory bulb (responsible for smell and taste), amygdala (responsible for emotions and moods), hippocampus (which processes and stores short-term memory), pituitary and pineal glands (which help regulate hormones), and thalamus (which acts as a switching station, routing messages into and out of the "higher" brain).

The midbrain's glands and bodies sit on top of the brain's stem, or spinal nerve, and cerebellum. The brain stem, besides being the seat of control for your digestive, respiratory, circulatory, and other systems, becomes your spinal cord. Encased in the protective bones (vertebrae) of your spine, it reaches about two-thirds of the way down your back. The cerebellum, adjacent to the brain stem, is responsible for balance and physical coordination.

The brain and spinal cord, which make up the central nervous system, work in conjunction with the peripheral nervous system, a web of voluntary and involuntary nerves branching out from your brain (cranial nerves) and spine (spinal nerves). These nerves weave their way around all your bones and into and through every tissue and muscle in your body – right down to your fingertips and toes.

Most nerves contain two kinds of fibers. Sensory fibers carry messages from your skin, muscles, and organs to your brain. Motor fibers carry instructions from whichever layer of the brain responded to the message (often it's all the layers) back to your muscles, tissues, and organs. Many nerve fibers going to muscles are voluntary, meaning that you have some conscious control over how they act. However, those going to and from glands and organs are part of what's called the autonomic nervous system; they work on their own. And that's a good thing. No one could consciously coordinate *all* the systems and processes needed to maintain life for five minutes, much less 24/7.

As command central for your body, your brain takes in thousands of bits of information per second, collates and analyzes it, compares it to and integrates it with previously gathered and stored information, and uses what it comes up with to generate a response.

Sometimes – such as when you pull your head out of the way of an oncoming fist – they're split-second responses, and as you throw a return punch or turn tail and run, they often lead to split-second reactions.

Other times, they're things you've mulled over at length: Shall I marry Harry or David?

Normal aging of the brain

Now that you've got a bit of brain biology under your belt, let's talk about how the brain matures and ages, both normally *and* abnormally.

Despite research conducted in the late 1980s, which showed that adult human brains can grow new cells (specifically in the olfactory bulb and hippocampus), most people have all the brain cells they're ever going to have by the time they're in their early 20s. And the number of nerve cells in the brain decreases from then on. By age 85 or 90, brain size and weight have declined by as much as 10 percent. In some areas of the brain, such as the brain stem, cell loss is meager; in others, such as the midbrain's hippocampus, it is pronounced.

Brain Myth #1: The brain powers down as you age.

In one sense, it's true. Brain-cell function does slow as you age, and it does become more difficult to store and retrieve things from short-term memory. But like good wine, aging can also make a well-used brain better. As you age, your brain cells build stronger and better connections, which means that as you experience events, you can do more crosslinking, cross-indexing, and cross-connecting. And as you age, the practice, experiences, and insights gained over time come into play in entirely new and creative ways.

As you age, fat starts getting deposited in brain cells and in the blood vessels feeding the brain. Free oxygen radicals, which tend to gum things up, begin accumulating around cells. Decline occurring in the bodies and glands of the midbrain has an impact on the levels and strength of the hormones and neurotransmitters that they and the cortex produce. Blood flow to the brain decreases by 20 percent; it decreases more if people have diabetes, high blood pressure, or heart disease. The number of cells in the spinal cord dips a bit, and nerve response decreases in organs, on the skin, and in the extremities.

What this adds up to cognitively and physically is that around the time you hit 60 (earlier if you haven't kept in good physical shape), brain function and physical coordination start a slow decline. It takes a bit longer to remember a word or name or where you left the car keys, or to decide whether to wear the red tie or the green one. It takes you a bit longer to feel pain, heat, cold, or pressure, or to catch your balance if you slip.

"A bit longer" is the key phrase here. Something that took five minutes to do at 60 takes you five minutes and ten seconds to do at 62, five minutes and twenty seconds at 65. You get the picture.

People who are aging healthily don't even notice most of these changes until their 70s, because the shifts occur so gradually that they don't interfere with quality of life. In fact, if they do take place rapidly enough for you to notice them, that's a red flag that something is wrong.

Optimal brain aging

That said, a healthy brain still has the ability to change and grow throughout its life span. It does that by adding dendrite branches to form more connections with other cells and by maintaining a high level of neurotransmitter production. The more you use your brain by challenging it and stimulating it with cognitive and physical activities, the more dendrites the brain cells make, enabling more connections to be made and more neurotransmitter cells to be sent out.

Researchers have found that sprouting more dendrites and making more brain-cell connections doesn't just increase experience, knowledge, and insight (and maybe even intelligence). It alters and improves mental health, too. That's because production of "feel-good" hormones, such as serotonin, increases when you participate in an activity that gives you "success." But more important, they have found that growing more dendrites and making more brain cell connections increases brain "plasticity" and "redundancy." That means that as you age, your brain is able to maintain optimal function because it is able to call on more cells to do a job or it is able to use different cells or combinations of cells to do it.

Brain Myth #2: The older you get, the more inflexible your personality becomes.

A study of women in midlife and beyond who had been tracked by the same psychologist since 1958 found that "affect optimization" (the ability to rein in one's less attractive personality traits and highlight the better ones) and "affect complexity" (the ability to evaluate and use conflicting data and information objectively) came to full flower in the women's 50s and 60s. So did their ability to handle ambiguity and manage relationships. In effect, what the study showed is that as we age, our temperament can "reorient" or become more relaxed and more flexible as we gain knowledge, experience, and insight.

An example of the plasticity/redundancy principle is a computer printer. In order to print a page, your computer processing unit ("brain") sends an electronic message ("neurotransmitter") to the printer. The message can be sent by the print function in the pull-down menu, or by either the Alt P or Print Screen keys. All get the job done the same.

Research is beginning to show that the plasticity/redundancy principle may also mean that you can build up cognitive brain "reserves" (as you can build calcium reserves for your bones) that you can take into very old age with you. One study, conducted with a group of nuns, showed that, at autopsy, the brains of several of the extremely active nuns all had the classic signs of brain damage due to Alzheimer's disease, yet while they lived they exhibited *none* of its symptoms. That means that for all intents and purposes, they didn't have Alzheimer's.

But that's how a brain ages at its physical and cognitive best. All brains don't age normally.

Abnormal aging of the brain, as well as the physical, mental, and psychological decline that comes with it, is due to primary or secondary diseases that irreparably damage or destroy brain cells and tissue.

Primary diseases are neurodegenerative diseases or conditions that arise in the brain and destroy brain cells. The most common in middle-aged people is multiple sclerosis. In older people, primary conditions include Alzheimer's disease, Parkinson's disease, Pick's disease, or Lewy body disease. Secondary conditions include vascular disease, brain tumors, and cancer. Cancer can be both a primary and secondary cause of brain damage and cognitive decline. Some people who develop lung cancer produce a substance that affects the brain so that it sends faulty messages promoting profound weakness out to the muscles. Ovarian cancer can produce a neurotransmitter that impairs concentration, focus, and the ability to carry out normal daily activities.

Brain-cell destruction that doesn't originate in the brain tissue itself is the second major cause of abnormal brain aging and cognitive decline. It can be due to past head trauma (think of Muhammad Ali); fluid buildup in the brain (normal-pressure hydrocephalus); long-term alcohol or substance abuse; viral infections, such as AIDS or syphilis; radiation therapy to the head; and nerve-damaging chemotherapy or medications. A recent study conducted by the National Institute on Aging added a high systolic (top number) blood pressure in *midlife* to the list of brain-cell destroyers.

It's not always bad news

The good news here is that in some situations, what looks like brain-cell destruction and cognitive decline in older adults isn't always. Many people who show symptoms of confusion, forgetfulness, and extremely slowed responses and reaction times need hearing aids or glasses. Once their vision and hearing are corrected, they return to normal.

Others are dealing with a thyroid dysfunction or nutrient deficiency (Vitamin B_{12}, folic acid, protein, niacin, etc.) that causes the symptoms. Some are abusing alcohol or taking medications that cause symptoms such as memory loss, confusion, agitation, slurred speech, falls, etc., which mimic cognitive decline. Still others are battling severe depression, which causes many of the same symptoms – weight loss, anxiety, anger, social withdrawal – of cognitive decline. The older the person, the more likely that these factors are causing or contributing to cognitive decline. (*See Memory-Robbing Medications, page 84.*)

The additional good news is that all can be reversed with proper diagnosis and treatment!

However, where there is severe depression, recovery may not be permanent. In the elderly, severe depression is often triggered by physical changes in the brain. It can also precipitate them. Even though the cognitive function of a severely depressed person improves with medication and therapy (a combination of both seems to work best), a chance of nearly 50 percent exists that the individual will develop irreversible dementia within the next several years.

Brain Myth #3: Once brain cells are lost, they're gone forever.

Research carried out since the late 1980s has shown that not only can the brain make new cells (although it's yet to be demonstrated that they do anything), it can also "coax" other cells to take over the function of damaged or dead cells when they are stimulated and trained to do so. Recently, there has been an explosion in the number of research projects and programs on retraining the brain, which help people compensate for cognitive and functional loss by teaching them how to use different parts of their brains, training them to use all their senses to access the information stored in damaged cells, and teaching them "spaced retrieval" strategies that enable them to remember information for longer and longer periods. Many of these techniques are being developed and fine-tuned by people who conduct Alzheimer's research or who have themselves experienced profound cognitive loss. For instance, the Serper Method was developed by Lynn Lazarus Serper, who earned her doctorate after suffering a burst artery in her brain and a post-surgical brain stroke that left her severely cognitively impaired for five years.

The body-brain connection

With all the hype about cognitive and mental decline, people tend to overlook the fact that whether you're 40 or 60 or 80, you aren't going to keep your wits about you as you age unless the rest of your body is in good physical health, too. And it's never too late to start putting that house in order!

First on the list to better brain health is to maintain a healthy weight. Being overweight increases your blood pressure and puts you at increased risk for diabetes. Both conditions put your brain at risk for infarcts (brain strokes) and other circulation-related brain-cell destruction.

Also, rethink how you eat. For good physical *and* brain health, eat four or five small meals a day rather than three larger ones. Spreading meals out helps your body remain on an even keel throughout the day and assures your brain of a continuous supply of nutrients, rather than a morning peak, a noon peak, and an evening peak. Along with the peaks come the valleys, which often lead to an insulin-induced drop in blood sugar (hypoglycemia). This can cause anxiety, mood swings, and nervousness, and lead to snacking on junk food.

Next up, do whatever it takes to achieve and maintain good heart, lung, and circulatory function. Oxygenated blood must circulate in the brain under normal pressure if the brain is to maintain its health. Activities that adversely affect your heart, lungs, arteries, or veins (such as the consumption of high-fat foods, smoking, and maintaining a sedentary lifestyle) will also adversely affect your brain. Sometimes, as with a heart attack that cuts off blood to the brain, the effect is immediate. At other times, as with the tiny and often unnoticed brain strokes that come with vascular dementia (the second most common form of dementia after Alzheimer's), it's cumulative.

In addition, make sure that chronic conditions such as diabetes, arthritis, or gum disease are properly treated and controlled. This "secondary prevention" pays big dividends. Studies suggest but don't prove that there are lower rates of Alzheimer's disease among diabetics with good blood-sugar control, arthritis patients who are taking nonsteroidal anti-inflammatory drugs (i.e., aspirin, ibuprofen, or naproxen), and people who have good oral health. And make sure that conditions causing chronic pain, such as osteoarthritis or fibromyalgia, are treated early and aggressively. A recent study showed that patients who endured chronic pain lost brain mass; the amount lost correlated with the duration of the pain.

Along with taking care of chronic conditions, take care of your immune system and your nervous system by eating nutrient-dense foods (*see Chapter 3: Eating for Life*). Both help the body fight off infections and diseases that could affect brain health, and both are constantly repairing themselves. If you aren't eating the right foods, you aren't providing the immune and nervous systems with the materials they need to do their jobs or make repairs. The immune system needs lots of protein and antioxidants. The nervous system, especially the brain, requires lots of carbohydrates and essential fatty acids. While your arteries don't need fat, your brain cells' axons do (for the myelin sheath covering them), so don't skimp on this very important dietary component.

Brain Myth #4: The major cause of memory impairment is dementia.
Research performed at the University of Kentucky's Sanders-Brown Alzheimer's Disease Research Center showed that only about 5 percent of all memory dysfunction can be laid at the door of dementia. Lack of adequate sleep; hearing and vision problems; depression, grieving, and stress; a chronic condition, such as diabetes or heart disease; drug or alcohol addiction; medication reactions and interactions; and lack of exercise cause more memory impairment than do irreparably damaged brain cells.

There are good observational studies suggesting that certain antioxidants – Vitamin E, Vitamin C, lycopene, etc. – may protect the brain and nervous system against some kinds of dementia *and* slow the progression of symptoms of early dementia. If you can slow progression so that you don't show signs till you're 90, and you die at 85, you have in effect *prevented* dementia.

There are also good studies that indicate that certain B vitamins (B_6, B_{12}), zinc, and folic acid may play a role in maintaining the health of the brain and nervous system. In fact, you can't go more than a month without feeling the effects, such as confusion and memory impairment, of folic acid deficiency. Some observational studies have also shown that folic acid deficiency is not only a risk for cognitive decline, it's a risk for heart disease, too.

A recent study found that moderate alcohol consumption also contributes to brain (and heart) health, at least if you're female and over 70. The study tracked the drinking habits of more than 12,000 women and found that those who drank the daily equivalent of a 12-ounce bottle of beer, a 4-ounce glass of wine, or a shot-and-a-half of whiskey (about 15 grams of alcohol) had a higher cognitive score than nondrinkers or those who consumed more alcohol. They also had a 20 percent lower risk of cognitive impairment as well as a significantly lower risk for cognitive decline. Researchers speculated that the benefit derived from alcohol may be indirect: It may preserve vascular function in the brain, which might prevent strokes and brain-cell destruction.

And finally, a growing number of studies show that getting adequate sleep – at least seven or eight hours a night – is a prime requisite for good brain (and mental) health. Sleep gives the brain and the cardiovascular system necessary downtime for repairs, rejuvenation, and rest. (There's a 20 to 30 percent drop in blood pressure and a 10 to 20 percent drop in heart rate during sleep.) It's the time when the brain produces and then circulates many of the hormones regulating the body's circadian rhythms, and it allows the brain to process and solidify experiences, memories and newly learned lessons. This is probably why, when you "sleep on it," you often tend to come up with an insight or a solution to a problem.

How to maintain healthy thoughts and emotions

Once you've laid the physical foundation for good brain health, the next step is to do the same thing for good cognitive and emotional health, which often go hand in hand. Below are some of the more important steps to take.

■ Hit the books early and often. Research shows that people who have the most education, whether they get it in the classroom or through self-directed reading, also tend to show the least measurable cognitive decline and have the lowest incidence of all forms of dementia. Researchers haven't identified exactly why this occurs; however, the most generally accepted hypothesis is that educational activities may be stimulating the brain cells to sprout more dendrites. The more dendrites a cell has, the more they're able to "talk" to each other. The more they talk, the more plasticity, redundancy, and brain reserve the brain has. This leads to greater cognitive health, now and in the future.

■ Become a lifelong learner. This is the other side of hitting the books. As you age, if you stay engaged – at your job, with a hobby, in volunteer activities, by enrolling in classes, by socializing and traveling, by taking on tasks that are challenging and stimulating – you're banking a cognitive reserve that you can draw on in your 70s and 80s. This cognitive reserve has the potential to push cognitive decline and function-robbing dementia right out of the picture.

■ Exercise your brain. No matter what your age, if you "brainercize," which means participating in stimulating activities that keep your brain cells firing on all pistons, the brain is in better shape to respond when it's called upon, and so are you.

An example of that is what I call the noradrenalin response. The stimulation of engaging in interesting activities such as doing a crossword puzzle, listening to a jazz CD, taking a t'ai chi class, piecing together a quilt, or coordinating the community food drive increases the release of neurotransmitters, especially norepinephrine, which is involved in alertness and attention. The norepinephrine makes it easier for you to stay focused during the activity, grasp concepts and ideas, assimilate information, and respond to it appropriately. Return to the task the following day, and things get even easier.

This kind of repetition has a very positive carry-over effect. Each time you participate in the activity that stimulates the release of norepinephrine, you deepen and strengthen brain-cell connections, and reshape and remodel your brain to respond more quickly and effectively to similar situations. And you're creating an environment in which "aha!" moments or sudden insights can take place.

■ Get physical. For decades, researchers have known that physical exercise and participating in pleasurable activities that require exertion and movement have a twofold effect on the brain.

When you participate in a strenuous exercise or activity that gets your heart rate up and your lungs pumping, circulation gets revved up. When more pressure is applied to your blood vessels, they open up and send more blood into the brain. This also allows individual brain cells to be flooded with oxygen and brain food (glycogen), so they work better and more efficiently. And brain cells pump out more of the "feel-good" hormones such as serotonin that de-stress the body, improve mood, and promote an overall sense of well-being – the well-known "exercise high." When you're participating in pleasurable activities, even ones that don't raise the heart rate, the same kinds of hormones are produced, just not so many. And the more often your brain cells produce those hormones, the better the prognosis for your current and future cognitive health.

■ Socialize. People who get out and about, who have a wide and varied social network, and who participate in both structured and unstructured group activities stay sharper longer. Recent research indicates that participating in intergenerational activities, such as tutoring in after-school programs or caring for grandchildren, may do the same thing. Many people have been heard to say, "My grandkids keep me young," so there may indeed be a cognitive benefit to pairing the old and the young.

■ Cut yourself some slack. After 60 or so, it gets more difficult to learn a new task – memorize names, follow directions for taking a new medication, program that new cordless phone – and retain newly learned information, because you've become more easily distracted and your response and reaction times have slowed. However, along with the drawbacks of slowing down there are benefits: the accumulated experiences, education, knowledge, understanding, and insight that have been encoded in the brain as wisdom, especially the wisdom to look into the mirror, see yourself as you are, and accept yourself and your circumstances with patience and grace.

Does "Brainercizing" Prevent Dementia?

The jury is still out on whether there is an actual cause-effect relationship between exercising the brain and the maintenance of cognitive health and performance in the elderly. While research does support the fact that using your brain improves your ability to use it in subsequent similar situations, no published studies have shown that taking on a challenging or stimulating task changes the structure (neuroanatomy) of the brain. What we do have is evidence – from real-time brain scans – that activities that are stimulating and challenging, such as solving math problems, reading poetry, and listening to complex music, increase glucose and oxygen use as well as neurotransmitter activity in the brain's outer layer (cortex).

It may be that people who already have good brain health and cognitive function are more likely to engage in the stimulating and challenging activities that tend to ward off cognitive and mental decline in old age. However, that doesn't mean that down the road we won't have proof – supplied by brain biopsies of individuals who "brainercized" their way into old age – that exercises and activities that make you think also help you keep your wits about you. Stay tuned on this one.

Ten tips and tricks for maximizing memory

It's a given: Your brain slows down as you age. It gets tougher to learn new things and to recall old information – what we call memory. This may be due to the fact that several of the areas of the brain that are responsible for information processing, sorting, and transfer to and retrieval from long-term memory tend to lose brain cells at an accelerated rate as you age or experience long-term chronic pain.

These ten tips won't just help you maximize memory and learn better; they'll also go a long way toward taking the stress out of your life.

- Actively gather information. Just because you listen to something doesn't mean you hear it; just because you notice something doesn't mean you see it. The best way to actively gather information is to immediately associate new information with something you already know or to put it into a context that you'll remember: how you'll use the new information, when you'll use it, etc.
- Use memory cues. Make lists. Record appointments and activities on a calendar and post it in a prominent place so that it's a constant visual reminder. Put Post-it notes on the bathroom mirror. Put the books that need to be returned to the library near the door to the garage. Use visual associations – for Mr. Katz, a cat; for Miss Smith, a horseshoe (remember when blacksmiths made horseshoes?) – to remember names.
- Gather and process new information with as many senses as possible. For instance, if you're programming that new cordless phone, don't just read the instructions. Get a feel for it with three of your senses: Hold it in your hand while you read the programming instructions out loud to yourself.
- Tune out distractions. As you age it gets progressively harder to focus, concentrate, and do more than one thing at a time.
- Break information into tasks or steps. If you're dealing with numbers or music, try learning backward – i.e., learning the last step first, then the next to last step, and so on. This may make the process faster and easier.
- Review what you want to remember. Some folks call this practicing. Teachers call it reinforcement.

- Habitualize. Becoming a creature of habit has two payoffs: You don't have to spend time wondering where the keys, glasses, or TV remote are, and you decrease stress and anxiety levels, too.
- Sleep on it. For many of the chemical changes to take place that turn data and experiences into long-term memory, the brain cells need downtime.
- Reduce your stress. No matter what your age, stress interferes with your ability to concentrate, stay focused, and remember things.
- Breathe. Lack of oxygen makes you tired and interferes with your brain cells' ability to take in, process, integrate, and store information. Practice sitting up straight and taking five deep, lung-filling, slowly exhaled breaths.

Spotting the red flags

It often begins with the car keys. Forgetting where you left them could be due to lots of things: work-related stress, fatigue from lack of sleep, too much wine, an adverse reaction to a blood-pressure medication, or your grief over a spouse's or friend's death. Or – if you're in your 60s – it could be an early sign of dementia, the insidious death of brain cells that eventually leads to memory loss, behavior changes, functional decline, multisystem shutdown, and death.

About 1 percent of the population between 60 and 64 shows signs of dementia. However, the incidence doubles every five years after that. By age 85, estimates are that half of those living on their own show some degree of dementia, and so do up to 80 percent of those living in nursing homes. The most common forms of dementia are Alzheimer's disease and vascular dementia. Together they make up about 90 percent of all dementia cases.

While the most common early symptom of dementia is forgetfulness, it's not *occasional* forgetfulness; it's constant forgetfulness and a host of other signs and symptoms.

Dementia is a progressive condition. In the early stage, symptoms may be mild, and people can often compensate for them and live on their own. As it progresses, however, symptoms become more pronounced, and the person usually needs round-the-clock care.

Generally, dementia causes the following signs and symptoms, which escalate in incidence and severity as the condition progresses.

■ Memory loss. Especially short-term memory loss that leads to repetitious questioning, misplaced possessions, and getting lost. As it progresses, it increases in frequency and intensity, and often causes anger, frustration, and paranoia. Because memory loss can affect the circadian rhythm, it may also affect or disrupt sleep, diet, grooming, and self-care patterns.

■ Problems with language. Initially, word-finding problems are solved with elaborate circumlocution: "You know, that thing with steps that goes up and down at the department store." In the final stage, ability to communicate verbally is lost.

■ Changes in personality. Mood swings and uncharacteristic social withdrawal or erratic behavior that slides into anger, hostility, or emotional unresponsiveness characterize early-stage dementia. As time passes, changes escalate and there is often deep depression or combative behavior. Since medications do slow the progression of some kinds of dementia, this is often the stage at which medical help is sought.

■ Disorientation. Those with early-stage dementia can often get along on their own, but as the condition progresses, they tend to misread and misinterpret their environment and become disoriented and confused about time and place.

■ Disruptive behavior. In the early stage of dementia, or when the person is in well-known surroundings, inappropriate and disruptive behaviors are at a minimum. Later stages, however, are usually defined by wandering, verbal abuse, physical aggressiveness, and other inappropriate behaviors (such as swearing, masturbating, or disrobing in public).

■ Inability to plan and carry out activities. While many people live on their own during the early stage of dementia, as it progresses, there is a steady decline in ability to manage finances, bathe and dress, prepare meals, and carry out activities of daily living.

A cognitive evaluation – yes or no?

Unless there is an underlying cause – trauma to the head, a brain tumor, long-term alcohol abuse, major depression – cognitive function is usually not affected until well into old age. When problems do arise, the most common cause is brain-cell destruction due to dementia, usually arising from Alzheimer's disease or vascular dementia.

A basic assessment of cognitive function can be done in a fifteen-minute office visit. Most family-practice physicians and internists as well as all geriatricians have a variety of tools available for generalized testing. The most-used "screens" are the Clock Drawing Test, the Mini-Mental State Examination (MMSE), and the Short Portable Mental Status Questionnaire (SPMSQ). In addition, since late-in-life depression is a red flag for cognitive decline, the Geriatric Depression Scale (GDS) is often used.

Generalized tests, are just that – generalized. They may indicate cognitive dysfunction, but that is not the same as dementia. A diagnosis of dementia requires documentation of a decline in intellectual function sufficient enough to *interfere with personal or occupational functioning.*

If scores are in the indeterminate range and the doctor has ruled out other causes – such as a brain tumor, adverse reactions to medication, dietary deficiency, etc. – the doctor may conduct a more comprehensive exam or refer the patient to a geriatric specialist, neurologist, or geriatric assessment center at a local hospital or university.

This second evaluation often requires more than one office visit because it thoroughly assesses ability to use language appropriately and follow verbal and written directions, place-time orientation, attention and recall of short-term and long-term memory, abstract thinking, insight into current health status, ability to navigate space, ability to solve math and visual problems, and mood and mental-health status. Because it is so thorough, this evaluation can sometimes identify the type and stage of dementia, but more important, it provides information and insights to shape the direction future decisions should take, and it provides patients and family members with information on interventions and resources that can help them plan for the future, manage change and maintain a satisfying and active quality of life.

Introducing MCI

In 2001, the American Academy of Neurology added a new category to the definition of dementia: mild cognitive impairment. In one sense, if you're going to become cognitively impaired, this is the condition to get.

Those with MCI are more forgetful than is normal for their age and health status. Indeed, memory problems are the chief defining characteristic of the condition. And they find learning new things harder than those without MCI. They usually need to use cues – written reminders, calendars, posted notes – so that everything that needs doing gets done. However, they still retain the thinking, reasoning, language, and social skills needed to be able to handle mild-to-moderately complex tasks, function on their own, and carry out activities – shopping, meeting friends for lunch, driving, playing golf – that allow them to retain their independence at home or in a setting that has been modified or chosen to meet their needs.

Many geriatricians believe that MCI is actually the earliest stage of Alzheimer's disease, one that we have only recently begun to be able to assess with tests and diagnose. And there may be some truth to that. About 40 percent of those who are diagnosed with MCI go on to develop Alzheimer's disease within five years, and almost all get the disease eventually.

Treatment recommendations vary because there is not enough long-term evidence about what may work to slow the progression of the condition. In most cases, physicians regularly monitor the person with MCI for changes in memory, thinking, and function that indicate worsening of the condition.

A three-year study published in *The New England Journal of Medicine* in 2005 may offer some hope for those diagnosed with MCI. It demonstrated that treatment with 10 milligrams of Aricept (donepezil) could delay the transition from MCI to Alzheimer's disease for about a year. However, delay is the key word here. By the end of the trial, the incidence of progression to Alzheimer's disease was the same for those who'd taken Aricept as for those who'd taken vitamin E (which showed no protective effect) and the dummy pill (placebo).

The Many Causes of Dementia

While amyloid clusters (gummy plaques) and short-circuited neurofiber masses (tangles) of Alzheimer's disease are responsible for the greatest number of dementia cases, as you will see from the following list, dietary deficiencies, injuries, diseases and conditions, and infections are also responsible for many of the situations that lead to dementia.

Metabolic-Toxic

Anoxia

B_{12} deficiency

Chronic drug-alcohol-nutritional abuse

Folic acid deficiency

Hypercalcemia associated with hyperparathyroidism

Hypoglycemia

Hypothyroidism

Organ-system failure
•Hepatic encephalopathy
•Respiratory encephalopathy
•Uremic encephalopathy

Pellagra

Structural

Alzheimer's disease

Amyotrophic lateral sclerosis

Brain trauma (acute severe)
•Chronic subdural hematoma
•Dementia pugilistica

Brain tumor

Cerebellar degeneration

Communicating hydrocephalus

Huntington's disease (chorea)

Irradiation to frontal lobes

Multiple sclerosis

Normal-pressure hydrocephalus

Parkinson's disease

Pick's disease

Progressive multifocal leukoencephalopathy

Progressive supranuclear palsy

Surgery

Vascular disease
•Multi-infarct dementia

Wilson's disease

Infectious

Bacterial endocarditis

Brain abscess (selective)

Creutzfeldt-Jakob disease

Gerstmann-Sträussler-Scheinker disease

HIV-related disorders

Neurosyphilis (general paresis)

Tuberculous and fungal meningitis

Viral encephalitis

Memory-Robbing Medications

It's a given that people over age 65 are prescribed more medications and more combinations of medications than someone younger. It's also a given that, due to the physical changes that take place as people age, a medication that works well for a 45-year-old with a hardy digestive tract and robust circulatory system isn't going to provide the same health benefits for a 75-year-old with ulcers and a tricky ticker. So it's also a given that many older adults – particularly those between 65 and 79 – show many of the signs and symptoms of early or mid-stage cognitive decline or dementia because the medications they're taking are poorly metabolized, poorly absorbed, or given in too strong a dose.

A panel of twelve geriatric, psychiatry, and pharmacology experts, convened by the Medical College of Georgia, the University of Georgia, and the pharmaceutical company Merck & Co., identified forty-eight individual medications or classes of medications that older adults should avoid.

For older adults, the following categories (with examples noted) tend to cause the most signs and symptoms of cognitive decline, including memory impairment, confusion, lethargy, withdrawal and depression, and in some cases agitation and seizures.

- Antihistamines, such as Benadryl or Chlor-Trimeton

- Muscle relaxants and antispasmodics, such as Robaxin or Paraflex

- Narcotic analgesics, such as Demerol or Darvon

- Long-acting benzodiazepines, such as Dalmane or Valium

- Tricyclic antidepressants, such as Elavil or Tofranil

- Antiemetics, such as Phenergan or Polaramine

- Gastrointestinal antispasmodics, such as Bentyl or Librax

- Histamine 2-receptor blockers, such as Tagamet or Zantac (at high doses)

In every instance, these medications and the others in their category have far less risky alternatives.

Chapter 7
Making Sense of Your Senses

When 77-year-old Adele P. showed up in my office with a huge mottled bruise snaking up her arm, I knew she was worried. She's not the kind of patient who comes in with twinges and dings – not even big dings.

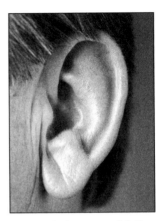

Adele explained that she was there because of two recent accidents: Two weeks ago she'd backed her car into another car in the parking lot at her bank. "The owner said he honked and honked, but I didn't hear him," she said.

Three days later, while grocery shopping, she'd lost her balance and fallen against a frozen-food case, which was where the bruise she was sporting had come from.

"It wasn't the store's fault that I fell," she said. "When he was helping me up, one of the people from the store told me that he'd called out to me not to go down the aisle because someone had just spilled milk. I heard him, but I didn't understand what he said.

"And," she added, "that's been happening for a while. If people aren't talking directly to me, or if the TV's not turned up, all I hear is mumbling or buzzing. And my ears ring a lot, but I don't notice that so much except at night when I'm trying to get to sleep."

A check of Adele's ear canal showed no buildup of wax or problems with her eardrum, and a quick review of her medication list and the supplements she'd been taking turned up nothing that could be causing a hearing loss. But her symptoms all pointed to it, so we set up an appointment with the audiologist.

When I saw Adele ten days later, the audiologist's tests confirmed my diagnosis: She had presbycusis, moderate, high-frequency hearing loss in both ears. In other words, she could "hear" sounds but not understand them.

When she asked what her options were, I was blunt. "Hearing aids or missing out on life for the rest of your life."

With guidance from the audiologist, Adele decided to go with a pair of digitally programmable in-the-ear hearing aids. Getting used to hearing again took time and perseverance. "The audiologist did a good job of programming my hearing aids," Adele said. "But it still took my ears a couple of months to get comfortable with them.

"But it was definitely worth the work," she added. "I just attended my 7-year-old granddaughter's first piano recital. She played *Für Elise*."

It just makes sense

René Descartes, the 17th-century French philosopher, said, "I think, therefore I am."

He was only partly right. What he should have said was "I have sensory organs that gather experiences and information that my brain processes and integrates so that I can understand the world I live in and make decisions, therefore I am."

I devoted a significant portion of the last chapter to talking about brain health, cognitive health, and psychological health, as well as how intertwined they are and how important it is to keep all three stimulated, challenged, and motivated.

This chapter is about keeping your sensory equipment (the organs that keep your brain informed, stimulated, and challenged) healthy and firing on all pistons.

But before we do that, let's talk about why you should keep your senses in tiptop shape.

■ Quality of life. Your senses are key components of your physical, social, psychological, and emotional health. You use them to gather the information that informs every decision you make. To move – sit, stand, walk, bike, catch yourself as you trip – you use your senses. To communicate and socialize and maintain good relationships, you use your senses. But your senses don't just enable you to experience life; they enable you to enjoy it, too. There's a hedonistic value to being able to taste a great Chardonnay, smell the first rose of summer, hear the haunting flute melodies of a Jean-Pierre Rampal CD, take in the grandeur and beauty of van Gogh's "Starry Night," and skate rings around the twentysomething couples at the ice-skating rink.

■ Cognitive health and function. Your sensory organs are your interface with the world. Next to the brain, they (and the nerve bundles that connect them to the brain) are the most important organs in the body. They're constantly sending perceptions, observations, and information (data) from your environment to the brain. Once there, it is analyzed, interpreted, integrated with previously gathered information, and used immediately or stored for future use. In addition (as noted in the previous chapter), all those bits of incoming data stimulate brain cells to create more dendrites and send out more neurotransmitters, making them better able to interpret and process information now and in the future.

The brain and the senses are a linked system. One without the other is useless. That's one of the heartbreaking ironies of a stroke or dementia. The sensory organs look and work fine, their receptors take in and send sensations to the brain, but the brain's cells are so damaged that they can't read the message, or they misread it. The eyes of a 75-year-old Alzheimer's patient may correctly send a visual message to the brain that says, "Sunlight is passing through the tree branches outside the window and casting a shadow of barren tree limbs on the wall." But the brain's Alzheimer's-damaged visual cortex reads the message as "There is a dark and skinny monster climbing on the wall."

And the eyes aren't the only sense organs sending messages that get misread.

You lose it as you use it

Your sensory organs are there for the long haul. But, as you age, they do gradually dull. Hence there's a loss in the ability to distinguish different shades of the same color or to read fine print; to taste and smell the difference between an extraordinarily fine wine and a merely good one; to tolerate changes in heat and cold, or notice when you've been cut; to hear high- or low-decibel sounds; or to recover quickly when you trip on a step.

That sensory dulling is due, in almost every case, to two things: the gradual loss of receptors in the sensory organ itself and an infinitesimal slowing of the time it takes for the information sensed by the organ's receptors to reach the brain for interpretation.

In general, you reach your sensory peak in your 20s. Sensory decline begins taking place soon afterward, but it's so gradual that until you hit your 60s, you don't notice, for instance, that food is tasting blander or it's harder to hear what's being said in a crowded room.

Also, you unconsciously compensate for the changes. You add a little more salt to the soup or turn your head so that your ear is pointed directly at whoever is speaking. Or you may consciously compensate. You get glasses, or you ask people to speak up or repeat things.

When change isn't normal

Dulling of the senses is normal. Loss isn't. When you lose a sense, or it becomes so dulled that you become consciously aware of its decline, that's a red flag that something is wrong.

"Something" could be a disease or condition. Multiple sclerosis, diabetes, vascular disease, and high blood pressure can all affect the eyes. Smell and taste are both affected by kidney failure and glossitis (a disease of the tongue). Paget's disease can fuse the bones of the inner ear and cause hearing loss.

Or it could be an infection. Candidiasis, a yeast infection in the mouth and throat, can interfere with taste.

It could be a bad habit. Smoking plays havoc with smell and taste.

It could be a vitamin or mineral deficiency. People who don't have enough zinc in their diet can lose their sense of smell. Those who skimp on antioxidants (beta carotene, vitamins C and E, zinc, etc.) risk losing their sight to age-related macular degeneration.

Or it could be the side effect of a prescription or nonprescription medication. Many chemotherapy drugs cause loss of the sense of taste. ACE inhibitors, taken by many with heart and kidney disease, can cause loss of smell and taste. High doses of such medications as aspirin, Edecrin (a diuretic), and streptomycin (an antibiotic) can all cause hearing loss. Anticholinergic medications, such as Ditropan, Elavil, or Benadryl, can cause blurred vision and worsen glaucoma. In fact, because older adults are taking so many medications, and because medication use is often behind a sudden sensory loss or cognitive decline, people who are experiencing either or both conditions should have their medications (and supplements) reviewed by a physician.

Or, as mentioned above, it could be the result of a brain injury or dementing condition that interferes with how the brain processes the information that the sensory organs are sending.

Eyes: Your window on the world

The sensory organs that concern people most are their eyes, the windows to the world. Almost 80 percent of everything we know reaches our brain through our eyes.

The Eye Guys: Who Does What

Before you turn 50, you should see an eye doctor at least every three years. After that it should be every two years. You should go more often if you have a condition such as diabetes or hypertension that can damage the eyes.

Whom you consult, however, depends on what you're looking for and the state of health of your eyes.

Opticians follow prescriptions written by ophthalmologists and optometrists, and are responsible for fitting glasses (including frame selection) and contact lenses and for instructing clients in how to care for them.

Optometrists can provide most routine vision care. Using a variety of assessment tools and equipment, they test eyes for visual acuity (sharpness), depth perception (nearsightedness and farsightedness), field of vision (side vision), ability to focus and coordinate eye function, and color perception. They write prescriptions for eyeglasses and contact lenses and can also prescribe and administer medications used to treat common eye diseases, such as blepharitis (inflammation of the edge of the eyelid) and dry eye due to Sjögren's syndrome. While they can also test for astigmatism (eye-muscle function), glaucoma, and diabetic retinopathy, they must refer those patients to an ophthalmologist for treatment.

Ophthalmologists are medical doctors who have received additional and specialized training in eye care. They provide primary eye-care services similar to those provided by an optometrist, but they also perform surgical procedures, such as laser surgery to reattach a retina or lens-replacement surgery to restore sight to eyes blinded by cataracts. In addition, they provide care, including surgical and nonsurgical interventions, for patients with complicated eye diseases, conditions, and disorders of the eyes.

Sight isn't just about your eyes, however. Vision is a three-part system. It includes the eyeball, which gathers and focuses light on the retina, a concentrated layer of receptors at the back of the eyeball; the optic nerve bundle, which sends what the retina senses to the brain; and the visual cortex, at the back of the brain, which interprets the light signals transmitted by the optic nerve.

Normal age-related changes in the eye and vision usually start in your 40s with presbyopia, a hardening of the lens of the eye that makes focusing on objects closer than two feet difficult. A trip to the optometrist for reading glasses usually solves this problem.

As you continue aging, other normal changes occur. It becomes more difficult to see things in dim light and to distinguish colors, especially blue, because the lens of the eye yellows with age and the receptors on the retina become dulled. In most cases, you can address this issue simply by changing to light bulbs of a higher wattage.

Also, the muscles controlling the opening and closing of the pupils of the eye become weaker, so they react more slowly to sudden light changes. This is why, when you go from a dark room into a well-lit one or vice versa, it takes longer for your eyes to adjust.

Your field of vision decreases, which means that you become less able to track what's coming at you from the side. Recent research has shown that this is a major cause of accidents involving those 70 and older.

The tear (lachrymal) and oil (sebaceous) glands that produce lubricants for the eyeball's surface decrease production, which often leads to dry eye or irritations that cause infections.

The eye's appearance changes, too. A grayish ring (arcus senilis) may appear around the pupil, and the white of the eye (sclera) may become slightly yellowed, browned, or dotted with brownish splotches. Yellowish globs (xanthelasmas) may appear on the eyelids or around the eye. The muscles controlling the lids may weaken, allowing the upper lids to drop down and cover the eyeball (ptosis) and/or the lower lids to fall into it (entropion) or away from it (ectropion). In addition, the fat deposits in the eye's socket may shrink, causing the eyeball to settle deeper into the socket (enophthalmos).

Age-related changes are normal; eye *disorders* aren't. (*See The Vision Robbers, pages 91-92.*)

The Vision Robbers

Sight is the sense we fear losing the most. The following four disorders are responsible for more than 90 percent of all vision loss.

Cataracts are the most common. They're a progressive clouding of the lens of one or both eyes that dulls and blurs vision and eventually leads to vision loss. Smokers and those who have spent long hours in the sun are most at risk for cataracts. Running a close second are dark-eyed people, longtime corticosteroid users, those with uncontrolled diabetes, and those who have injured an eye in the past.

When vision is impaired by cataracts, glasses and better lighting can compensate for decades. When they're no longer effective, surgical removal (phacoemulsification) of the clouded lens, replacement with an artificial (intraocular) lens, and a new pair of glasses usually provide an acceptable level of vision. When lens implantation is not possible, contact lenses or thick eyeglasses often provide the same effect.

About 95 percent of surgeries result in improved vision. When problems (infection, bleeding, increased eye pressure, lens displacement) do occur, however, they often lead to blindness.

Glaucoma, the second most common eye disorder, is caused by an increase in the pressure of the fluid behind the eye's lens. There are two types: open-angle or chronic glaucoma, which is the more common, and closed-angle or abrupt-onset glaucoma. Left untreated, both damage the optic nerve and cause blindness.

Everyone over 60 is at risk for glaucoma. Those who are most at risk include people with a close (first-degree) relative with glaucoma or who have diabetes, African Americans and Asians, and people who have undergone long-term corticosteroid use. Symptoms are vague, with blurred vision and blind spots being the most common, so the only way to be sure that you don't (or do) have glaucoma is a visit to an ophthalmologist. The visit should include an eye-pressure check with a tonometer, an interior-of-the-eye scan with an ophthalmoscope, and a full field-of-vision test.

If glaucoma is diagnosed, the usual treatment for open-angle glaucoma is lifetime use of prescription eye drops or creams – such as Timolol or Brinzolamide – to control eye pressure. The usual treatment for closed-angle glaucoma is surgery or laser therapy to improve fluid drainage in the eye. Treatment may "cure" this form of glaucoma; however, regular monitoring of the condition is still needed.

Macular degeneration is the most common cause of blindness in people over 60. Like glaucoma, it has two forms: In the dry (nonvascular) form, the retina thins and the light-sensitive cells of its macula are lost; in the wet (vascular) form, leaky blood vessels grow on and under the retina, causing the macula area to wrinkle and scar.

Those most at risk include people with a family history of the disease, smokers, fair-skinned Caucasians, and those with a low dietary intake of antioxidants. The disease progresses so slowly and painlessly that people unconsciously compensate for its signs: blurred or distorted vision and a central-vision blind spot. Like glaucoma, macular degeneration must be diagnosed in an ophthalmologist's office. Usually this is done with an interior-of-the-eye scan using an ophthalmoscope. In some cases, however, results are inconclusive. When that occurs, fluorescein angiography, which uses an injected dye to get a better look into the eye, may be used.

The aim of treatment is to slow the progress of the macula's degeneration. For the wet form of the disease, laser treatment to obliterate encroaching blood vessels has shown some success in preventing the progression of the condition. There is no treatment for the dry form of the condition, though studies indicate that high doses of antioxidants may slow its progression. Patients should receive information on low-vision aids and groups that can share advice, encouragement, and coping strategies.

The fourth disorder, **diabetic retinopathy**, is a consequence of diabetes. It is caused by damage done to the retina by the blood vessels that nourish it. Under normal circumstances, that's all they do. When diabetes is present, however, the blood vessels grow erratically, sprouting weak veins that tear, break, and leak blood into the retina, which causes it to bulge and eventually tear itself away from the back of the eye.

Sometimes diabetic retinopathy announces itself with blind spots, floaters, and flashing lights, but in general, an ophthalmologist makes the diagnosis by scanning the interior of the eye with an ophthalmoscope. Treatment – usually laser surgery (photocoagulation) to obliterate and cauterize the abnormal blood vessels and/or reattach the retina to the back of the eye – usually stops progression of the condition and in some cases improves vision. However, without strict management of the diabetes causing the problem, it usually recurs.

Taking care of business

To maintain eye health, have your eyes checked periodically. The older you are, the more often you should have an eye checkup. After you turn 50, you should have an ophthalmological exam every three years; when you hit your 60s, have one every two years. If you're dealing with chronic conditions that increase the risk for eye disease, such as diabetes or high blood pressure, have an eye exam every year. Not only will an ophthalmologist be able to detect and diagnose diseases and conditions that cause vision loss, but he or she will also be able to prescribe medications and/or suggest interventions to slow their progression.

To protect your eyes from the effects of the sun's ultraviolet (UV) rays, use sunglasses and wide-brimmed hats. While there are no conclusive human studies about the effects of ultraviolet light on the eye, animal studies *are* conclusive: UV light irreparably damages the eye.

If you have a condition or disease that can cause or exacerbate eye damage, such as diabetes or high blood pressure, do what it takes to keep the condition under control.

Don't smoke. Smoking constricts the blood vessels nourishing the eyes, and the fumes from smoke contain eye irritants.

Eat for eye health. Research shows that high doses of certain elements – beta carotene, vitamins A and C, zinc – can prevent or lower your risk for some eye conditions, including macular degeneration.

José, can you hear?

Hearing, like vision, is a multipart system. The outer ear collects sound waves and funnels them down the ear canal to the middle ear, where the eardrum and bones (ossicles) condense the waves and send them to the inner ear. There, they cause receptors in the cochlea to vibrate and send electrical signals to the auditory nerve, which forwards them to the brain, where they're interpreted.

Hearing loss is the most common disability of aging. Almost 30 percent of 65-year-olds have hearing loss; it jumps to 50 percent by age 80.

The two major kinds of hearing loss are sensorineural hearing loss and conductive hearing loss.

By far the most common, sensorineural hearing loss is due to loss of sensitivity to sound. The major cause of sensorineural hearing loss is age-related dulling of the receptors in the ear's cochlea (presbycusis). But such circumstances as exposure to loud noises, a blow to the head, and medications that affect the auditory nerve also cause hearing loss. Ringing in the ears (tinnitus) is an early indicator of sensorineural hearing loss.

Conductive hearing loss occurs when the airwaves that carry sound can't get to the middle and/or inner ear. Major causes for conductive hearing loss include earwax buildup, perforation of the eardrum, damage to the tiny bones in the middle ear (otosclerosis), and head trauma.

By age 60, most people have both kinds of hearing loss. But it's usually so mild that it's difficult to spot. That said, however, there are red flags that can indicate a problem.

- Constant ringing in the ears (tinnitus)
- The need to turn up the TV or radio until the walls shake
- Difficulty hearing high-pitched sounds, especially the voices of women and children
- Difficulty discerning words that begin with the letters C, D, F, K, P, S, and T
- Difficulty following conversations in a crowded or noisy room unless you turn your head so that an ear is directly in line with the speaker
- Inappropriate responses in social situations (which, in some cases, are mistaken for confusion or cognitive impairment)

Hearing loss can be diagnosed by a physician, but to learn the type and degree of loss involved and the appropriate treatments, it's best to have an audiologist perform a hearing evaluation. Along with a medical history and medication review, this includes a thorough inner-ear exam, a tuning-fork test (to test both pitch and conduction), an audiometric test (for loudness, pitch, tone and frequency thresholds), and a speech-recognition test (to identify speech discrimination, perception, and reception thresholds). On the basis of all these findings, audiologists provide a diagnosis, suggest appropriate treatment, and offer information about where to find assistive listening devices, such as portable telephone amplifiers and low-high-volume phones.

Sometimes treatment is as simple as a prescription for hydrogen peroxide or mineral oil to dissolve wax and keep it from redeveloping in the ear canal. At other times it's a referral to an aural surgeon for further testing that could result in a cochlear implant or surgery to separate fused inner-ear bones. Most of the time, however, treatment means a hearing aid.

Hearing aids are fitted by an audiologist. All hearing aids are battery-powered, with microphones that pick up sound and an amplification system that augments it and sends it to the middle and inner ear, where the auditory nerves "sense" it and transmit it to the brain.

In size, hearing aids run the gamut from large mechanisms that rest behind the ear to tiny units fitted inside it. They come in three different models.

- Analog – The most common and least expensive type of hearing aid, they simply amplify sound.
- Digitally programmable – Along with amplifying sound, they allow tinkering with settings for pitch and decibel.
- Digital – Not only do these units amplify sound, but they can be programmed to automatically lower incoming sound, screen out background noise, and focus on the direction from which sound is coming.

In just about every trial of hearing aids that's been published, they've been shown to improve not only hearing but also quality of life. Despite such beneficial evidence, most hearing aids end up in dresser drawers.

People don't want to wear them because they're for "old people." They also are hard to manipulate, and not just by people with arthritis. However, the main reason people don't like them is that the first time they use a pair of hearing aids – and most people do need two – their brains are blasted with sound they haven't had to deal with for years.

If people just stuck it out through the period of adjustment, the brain's ability to handle all that "new" information would return. But people don't realize that, so after four of five days of sensory overload, the hearing aids go into the drawer.

A new generation of hearing aids

For 95 percent of people with age-related hearing loss (presbycusis), a hearing aid could improve both their hearing and social life. But many of those who would get the most benefit from hearing aids won't even consider them because they think their only option is two 4-ounce pieces of putty-colored plastic hanging behind their ears. This is no longer so.

Over the last ten years, there has been a revolution in hearing aids. They're more user-friendly. And they better amplify the sounds people want to hear (a grandchild's laugh, a mockingbird's song) and block the sounds they don't (clattering silverware in a restaurant, coughs and sniffles at a concert).

"Pocket" hearing aids and units that rest behind the ear (BTE), in the ear (ITE), and concealed in the ear canal (CIC) are all available at prices ranging from under $1,400 (a basic pair) to more than $7,000 (for a sophisticated pair). Batteries last much longer in the newer models, in some cases up to twice as long as they did five years ago.

The revolution in hearing aids is due to the miniaturization and computer-ization of all the gadgetry inside them. In fact, some models run on chips with processing power greater than the capacity of some computers. Chips don't just mean smaller and lighter-weight units with fewer buttons, dials, and remote controls; they also mean that hearing aids can be reprogrammed as the user's hearing changes.

No matter how good they are, though, they aren't new ears. This new generation of hearing aids has dramatically improved things, but they don't give you perfect hearing. And they don't work at all if you don't break them in.

Once you decide on a hearing aid, the transition will be smoother if you bear the following things in mind.

■ Expect to spend three weeks to a month getting used to wearing a hearing aid.

■ Get accustomed to wearing the aid gradually. For the first week, use it two or three hours a day; during the second week, add a few more hours; during the third week, aim for all day.

■ Practice focused listening. Turn on the TV or radio and have someone speak to you or read to you. As you concentrate on what they're saying, you'ill build up your ability to filter out background noises.

Holding hearing loss at bay

You can't prevent hearing loss, but you can take measures to put it off and lessen its impact when it does appear.

At the top of the list: Avoid loud noise and high-frequency sounds as you age. Both significantly damage the workings of the inner and middle ear.

Know your heredity risk for hearing loss. Some conditions, such as the fusing of the tiny bones of the inner ear (otosclerosis) and Ménière's disease, run in families.

Keep ear canals free of wax, and treat ear infections *promptly.*

Check your dental bite. Grinding your teeth, especially during sleep, can trigger jaw pain that becomes ear pain and ringing in the ears.

Monitor medications. Certain over-the-counter and prescription diuretics and analgesics increase the risk for hearing loss. In many cases, when you stop taking a medication, hearing problems disappear.

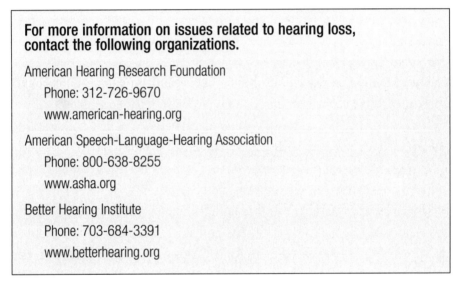

For more information on issues related to hearing loss, contact the following organizations.

American Hearing Research Foundation
   Phone: 312-726-9670
   www.american-hearing.org

American Speech-Language-Hearing Association
   Phone: 800-638-8255
   www.asha.org

Better Hearing Institute
   Phone: 703-684-3391
   www.betterhearing.org

The dynamic duo: Taste and smell

No two senses work more closely than smell and taste. Both are chemosensory senses, which means that their receptors sense and react to chemical molecules.

The organ for odor detection is the olfactory bulb. When you breathe air in through your nose, the odor molecules it contains travel up your nasal cavity and bounce off the olfactory bulb's receptors, which are covered in mucus. As a receptor absorbs an odor molecule, it sends a message to the olfactory bulb, which forwards it to the brain, where it is identified – "Skunk!" – and acted upon.

The tongue is the major organ for taste, but the soft palate and the gums play roles, too. All have receptors that react to the chemical molecules carried to them in saliva as you chew food and move it around in your mouth. When a receptor "senses" a taste, it sends a message to the glossopharyngeal nerve under the tongue, which forwards it to the taste centers in the brain, where it is identified – "Chocolate!" – and acted upon.

It's impossible to maintain a good sense of taste without also maintaining good oral health. Many taste receptors are in the gums, so gum disease (gingivitis) impairs the ability to taste. It also causes periodontal disease, loosening ligaments and bones that support and anchor the teeth. When teeth are lost, so is the ability to break food down in the mouth so that it can be mixed with the saliva and "tasted."

Usually your sense of smell and taste are working simultaneously. Taste receptors (buds) in the mouth give you the ability to distinguish the basics – "It's sweet," "It's meat." Olfactory receptors in the nose give you the ability to fine-tune things, to tell the difference between dark chocolate and milk chocolate or between beef and pork. But they work independently, too. If you have a disease that affects the glossopharyngeal nerve, you may not be able to taste food, but you can still distinguish and enjoy it with your sense of smell; if you lose your sense of smell, you can still enjoy foods through their temperature, texture (mouth appeal), and basic taste.

Though studies have shown that taste and smell receptors replace themselves, as you age, the number of taste and smell receptors declines, and so does the sensing ability of those that are left. Most people don't begin to notice these changes till their 60s (for smokers, it happens earlier). By age 75, however, about 40 percent of people report a significantly diminished sense of smell.

Gradual decline due to a dulling of receptors is normal; a rapid or sharp decline or a total loss of taste or smell is not. Both situations are red flags; you should see your family physician or an otolaryngologist (a physician specializing in diagnosing and treating ear, nose, and throat disorders).

When smell abruptly *declines*, there are a number of usual causes: nasal dryness, resulting from a decline in mucous production in the nasal passage; rhinitis, inflammation of the mucous membrane in the nose; sinusitis, inflammation of the sinuses due an allergic reaction or viral, bacterial, or fungal infection; or taking medications. Using a humidifier or saline nasal wash usually clears up nasal dryness. Topical nasal sprays and antibiotics usually work for rhinitis and sinusitis. Discontinuation of the drug or drugs causing the decline usually solves the medication problem. Antimicrobials, antihypertensives, diuretics, and vasodilators seem to be the worst offenders when it comes to medications that interfere with smell.

When smell is lost abruptly, it's usually due to head trauma, cancer, or a viral infection or flu that affects the olfactory receptors. In many cases, when people recover fully from the illness or injury causing a problem, their sense of smell does not. This is an important reason for older adults to get an annual flu shot and participate in exercise programs designed to prevent falls.

When ability to taste declines sharply, it's usually due to side effects from medications; poorly functioning salivary glands (xerostomia); tongue or gum disease; tooth loss and inability to chew; oral infections, such as thrush (candidiasis); or systemwide disorders, such as Sjögren's syndrome, hypothyroidism, or diabetes. In most cases, the sense of taste can be restored, although often not to its former level, through changing medications, addressing the cause of the salivary dysfunction (medications and surgery are common treatments), treating tongue or gum diseases, restoring ability to chew with dentures or implants, and treating the systemwide disorder causing the symptom.

Total loss of taste (ageusia) is rare. When it does occur, it's usually due to radiation or chemotherapy to treat cancer of the head or neck, a stroke affecting the taste center in the brain, or the effects of a dementing condition such as vascular dementia. In rare cases, it's also a symptom of psychotic, delusional depression.

No matter what the cause, however, a significant decline in or loss of ability to smell and/or taste should be treated as a significant medical condition, especially in the elderly, because such circumstances often lead to malnutrition and all the health problems that accompany it.

Maintaining oral health after 65

A generation ago, dentures were the norm for people in their 60s. Today, more and more older adults are taking the teeth they were born with into retirement with them.

The teeth of older adults have the same needs as those of the young. You have to floss them and brush them twice daily with plaque- and bacteria-fighting toothpaste.

But they have other concerns, too.

- **Sensitive teeth.** Older teeth have lost some of their protective enamel, so they're more sensitive to heat and cold. Avoiding extremely hot or cold foods and beverages, and using rinses and toothpastes with stannous or sodium fluoride often helps.

- **Dark teeth.** As noted above, older teeth have lost enamel, making the inner dentin more visible and also making it easier for the teeth to be stained by coffee, tea, and smoking. Whitening gels – applied at home or in the dentist's office – solve this problem nicely.

- **Breaking and chipping teeth.** Older teeth, both with and without fillings, are weaker and break more easily under pressure. Crowns restore both the look and the function of broken teeth.

- **Dry mouth.** The salivary glands become less productive, leaving teeth and gums at increased risk for buildup of tartar and plaque, gumline cavities, and cavities around the edges of old fillings. You can help keep saliva flowing by using artificial saliva, sucking on sugarless candy, or chewing sugarless gum.

- **Gumline cavities and periodontal disease.** Your gums recede as you age, leaving the roots of your teeth exposed to the cavity-causing effects of tartar and plaque as well as to the destruction of the ligaments and the bone that hold the teeth in place. Products containing additional fluoride help prevent gum problems.

- **Bad breath.** Medications, chronic conditions, and dry mouth are often responsible for bad breath. Use of an electric toothbrush, which allows for better reach and more thorough brushing, and brushing the tongue and inside the cheeks can often reduce or solve this problem.

- **Oral cancer.** About half of all cases of oral cancer occur in persons 65 or over. Regular visits to the dentist ensure early detection, which is the best defense against this aggressive and fatal form or cancer.

Touch: The body's armor

The skin is a three-layered wonder. The epidermis is made up of a layer of dead skin cells as well as an underlayer making the melanin that gives color to skin and the vitamin D that helps build strong bones and teeth. The dermis is composed of the connective fibers that give skin its strength and elasticity. This connective tissue is the matrix where the receptors for light touch, deep touch, heat, cold, and pain are found, as well as the sweat and oil glands and the hair follicles.

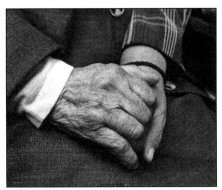

Just below the dermis, a fat layer acts as the body's insulation against cold and helps regulate the production and activity of certain hormones (including those that cause certain kinds of cancer). Also in this layer is the network of blood vessels that nourishes the other two layers.

When people think about aging and their skin, they think about wrinkles and sunspots and cancer, rather than the fact that the skin is their largest sensory organ, constantly feeding the brain information about the environment. It is also your body's armor.

When you're young, the dermis is a thick shield against cuts and agents such as chemicals and germs that could harm interior tissue and organs. In addition, the millions of receptors in the epidermis are at the peak of their performance. And the fat layer protects tissues and organs.

By your 60s, however, that changes. All three layers have become much thinner. Also, there has been a loss of sensory receptors in the epidermis, and the ability of the remaining ones to sense and respond to stimuli such as an icy car door, a hot pot handle, or a sharp pin has become dulled. And transmissions to the brain from those remaining receptors has slowed, too.

That one-two punch means that the skin shows slower response to adverse stimuli – burns, cuts, scrapes – and more vulnerability to red-flag situations that may not require a visit to the doctor but do require close monitoring. These include skin breaks that can come with dry, itchy skin; skin irritations from allergic reactions to such things as perfume or latex; friction-related problems, such as blisters and pressure sores; and conditions, rashes, and skin outbreaks such as rosacea (acne-like outbreaks) and psoriasis that encourage unconscious scratching.

In addition, because the body's armor is so easily "penetrated," the body is more susceptible to invasion by germs and microorganisms that attack organs or cause systemic infections. Because the fat layer that was protecting them has thinned, the risk for bruising and injury to capillaries, internal tissues, bones, and organs increases also. This is one of the major reasons that as you age you tend to bruise more.

Giving up smoking and tightly managing chronic conditions that affect circulation, such as diabetes, kidney disease, and heart disease, will help maintain the health of skin cells and tissues and nourish the sensors and nerves that connect skin to the brain.

Keeping the skin well moisturized by consuming plenty of water and applying products that contain high amounts of lactic or glycolic acid will help it maintain sensitivity to touch and pressure, and also help prevent minor skin breaks and itching. When skin outbreaks do occur, applying an antibiotic cream or lotion helps them heal faster and better. Certain conditions, such as psoriasis, also respond to light therapy (phototherapy).

Consuming foods rich in easily digested protein, omega 3 fatty acids, zinc, potassium, and vitamins C and E can also help keep all the layers of the body's biggest organ functioning at peak capacity.

The sixth "sense": Balance

Balance is equilibrium: knowing where you are in relation to the space you're in.

No single organ is responsible for balance, so it's not a sense. But it is the body's most sensory-dependent function.

Balance isn't a sensory function, however; it's a processing function. In order to maintain equilibrium, your brain is instantaneously receiving and integrating two kinds of sensory information from your ears: sonar-like readings that tell you where you are and directional readings from the fluid-filled balance organs in the inner ear that keep you oriented in terms of up and down, left and right, and front and back.

From your eyes, the brain is receiving, processing, and integrating visual cues that give it environmental information and line-of-sight readings that orient you as to distance, direction, obstacles, and speed. And the brain is receiving and processing information from the proprioceptors, special pressure nerves located in the soles of your feet and your muscles, tendons, and joints, which tell the brain precisely where and how you are standing and what each muscle, tendon, and joint is doing. It's also coordinating all this information so smoothly and effortlessly through both the central and peripheral nervous systems that you aren't even aware that thousands of tiny corrections – in everything from heel elevation to body sway – are being made to enable you to stand erect. Or take a step. Or turn a corner. Or step out of the way of an oncoming skateboarder.

The "sense" of balance begins to decline in your 40s, but decline is slow and gradual, and you do things to compensate for it such as walking with your toes pointed outward, so you don't realize that your balance and gait have changed until you're in your 60s. You only realize it then because you find it harder to right yourself when you trip on a crack, slip on the living-room rug, or "slide" through an intricate turn on the dance floor.

Every year, impaired balance causes falls in approximately 30 percent of people over the age of 65, and the incidence of falls increases with age. A fall that results in head trauma, a spinal fracture, or a broken hip can ground you for life.

Who's most at risk for falls?

- People with visual and hearing impairments
- Those with chronic conditions, such as alcoholism, arthritis, diabetes, or low blood pressure
- Those who are using over-the-counter sleep aids, antihistamines, and prescription-only medications for depression or seizures
- Those who are cognitively impaired
- Those who've become sedentary: This not only allows muscles in the back, legs, and ankles to get loose and flabby; it also contributes to "deconditioning" of the brain

While you can't prevent the age-related changes to your eyes, ears, and musculoskeletal system that contribute to loss of balance, it's definitely possible to prevent falls.

Since all your senses are nourished by and through the circulatory system, do what it takes to control the conditions like cardiovascular disease or diabetes that play havoc with the circulatory system.

Get into an exercise program that increases hip mobility and range of motion and strengthens leg muscles and joints. And do exercises (one-foot stands, side-to-side lunges, torso twists) that improve balance. Studies show that people who do flexibility and stretching exercises, especially t'ai chi, have fewer accidents and more physical confidence.

Take supplements that improve joint health, such as glucosamine, chondroitin, bromelain, and vitamin D.

And, since the overwhelming majority of falls take place in the home, fall-proof your house: Take up scatter rugs, install brighter bulbs in hall and stair fixtures, put up a grab bar in the bathroom, move often-used cookware to lower shelves, etc.

These changes don't just lower the risk of falls. Because they raise self-confidence, they boost quality of life, too.

Chapter 8
Senior Sexuality: You're Never Too Old for the Good Stuff

Sixty-seven-year-old Anthony P. first developed erectile dysfunction in his mid-50s. But it wasn't until a little over a year ago, when renovations had just started on his home and his wife, Carmella, was diagnosed with metastatic breast cancer, that loss of libido became a problem.

Indeed, it was during a lazy Sunday-afternoon session of what Anthony called "canoodling" that he noticed the lump in his wife's breast that sent her to the doctor. Six days later she underwent partial mastectomy and reconstructive surgery. Carmella is doing well with maintenance therapy, and the two just celebrated their 41st wedding anniversary. All the finishing touches have finally been added to the refurbished kitchen, family room, and deck as well.

But life hadn't righted itself. "I thought things would go back to normal when Mella got better and everything settled down at the house," Anthony explained. "But if anything, things have gotten worse. It's not just that I'm not interested in sex. I'm not interested in anything. I'm tired all the time."

Sex and the Senior Set: Myth #1

Myth: *Sex happens.*

Reality: Sex "happens" when you're a 19-year-old with nothing on your mind but sex. Given the complicated and hectic schedules most people are dealing with today, little time exists for the activities and intimacies that get your mind and body focused on sex – unless you make time for them. One way to do that is to designate one night a week (at least) as "date" night. An evening at the art museum, dinner with wine, a walk around the neighborhood at dusk – all can be the prelude to a pleasurable, intimate session behind closed doors.

A thorough physical, which Anthony was due for anyway, showed that his blood pressure and heart rate were normal, his lungs were good, and so were his testicles and prostate. His prostate was somewhat enlarged – a normal condition for a man his age – but there were no nodules. All his lab tests were normal, too, with the exception of his free testosterone level. At 1.2 (the normal range is 1.5-3.5) his lab results were noticeably below normal.

During his follow-up visit, I explained to Anthony that he wasn't dealing just with erectile dysfunction, an inevitable consequence of aging. He was also dealing with depression and low libido resulting from his low testosterone levels.

I explained that he had two options: a prescription for one of the pills made specifically for erectile dysfunction or testosterone supplementation. The former would improve blood flow to the penis and produce an erection, but it wouldn't address his other problems. The latter had the potential to improve his ability to get erections *and* boost his libido, energy levels, and sense of well-being, too.

Anthony went home with a trial prescription for a topical testosterone gel in his wallet and instructions to see me again in three months. The follow-up visit was needed because testosterone is a hormone, which could have an effect on his prostate, so I wanted to do a PSA test, and I wanted him to report back on how the gel was doing.

When Anthony returned for his check-up three months later, it was obvious that his life had finally righted itself. "Nothing happened for the first couple of weeks that I could notice. But one morning I woke up, and, well, we didn't get out of bed till past 10," a happy Anthony said.

Good sex is healthy

Senior sex is not an oxymoron. All the data available on people up to age 85 indicate that you're never too old to initiate, participate in, and enjoy sex. According to a survey commissioned by the National Council on Aging, not only are men and women in their 80s sexually active, but they report a high level of enjoyment and satisfaction, too.

The stress reduction and psychological benefits that come with an intimate and satisfying sex life are well known. Less well known are its health benefits. Sex burns calories (up to 150 a "workout"); the deep breathing and faster heart rate that are part and parcel of sexual intimacy increase blood flow to all organs; it helps lower levels of LDL, or bad cholesterol; it improves sleep; it dulls pain; it boosts levels of two main sex hormones, testosterone and estrogen; and, at least for men, it may promote a longer life. A report published in Great Britain in 2000 found that men who had more than two orgasms a week live longer than their less-orgasmic peers, and a 2004 study of almost 30,000 American men ages 46 to 81 showed that men who reported a lifetime history of twenty-one ejaculations per month had a significantly reduced risk for chronic prostate inflammation (prostatitis) and prostate cancer.

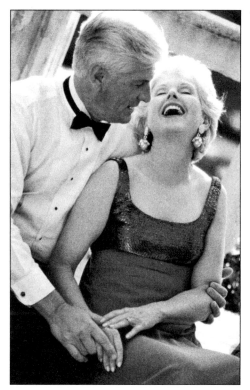

Hitting all the bases

Whether you're male or female, to be able to enjoy a satisfyingly intimate and sexual "encounter," you must go through all the emotional and physical phases of the sexual response cycle.

- **Phase 1: Excitement.** Interest is piqued through visual and physical stimulation; muscles tense; heart rate increases; blood flows to genitals, initiating lubrication of the woman's vagina, swelling of the man's penis, and production of male lubricating fluids and ejaculate.
- **Phase 2: Plateau.** Changes begun in Phase 1 go into overdrive; muscle tension peaks; whether through "outside" stimulation or vaginal penetration, the penis, clitoris, and vagina begin muscle spasms.
- **Phase 3: Orgasm.** Muscle spasms become contractions that forcefully release muscle tension built up in both partners and the ejaculate at the base of the penis.

■ **Phase 4: Resolution.** A general sense of intimacy and well-being engulfs both parties; heart and breathing rates return to normal as do swollen tissues. Women may experience further orgasmic activity; men require a recovery period before being able to reinitiate the cycle.

Sex and the Senior Set: Myth #2

Myth: *As women age, they lose interest in sex.*

Reality: The difference in the level of men's and women's sexual activity as they age has little to do with interest and desire and much to do with the availability of partners. Women typically outlive men – almost half of all women over the age of 65 are widowed or never married, while only 15 percent of men are – and they tend to survive into old age healthier, too.

Barriers to intimacy

While aging itself doesn't play a role in your ability to initiate and enjoy sex, the changes that take place in your reproductive organs do, and so does the effect those changes have on the sexual-response cycle.

Women have two sets of sex organs. The external genitalia include the labia, clitoris, Bartholin's (secretory) glands, and the opening to the vagina; internal genitalia encompass the vagina, uterus, cervix, fallopian tubes, and ovaries. Most of the changes that affect them come at menopause.

■ The sex drive (libido) may decrease, due to a drop in several sex-related hormones, including estrogen and testosterone.

■ During sexual arousal, the labia and clitoris are less engorged with blood.

■ The vagina lubricates more slowly, and the amount of lubrication decreases.

■ The tissue of the vaginal wall thins, leaving it more sensitive during intercourse.

■ The vaginal canal shortens, which can cause pressure and pain during intercourse.

■ The cervix (mouth of the uterus) and uterus shrink, which may lead to pain during intercourse, painful uterine contractions with orgasm, or less intense orgasms.

■ Rearousal after sex takes longer, or does not occur at all.

■ In addition, the drop in estrogen levels causes thinning and weakening of the lining and muscles of the urinary tract, which may lead to involuntary leakage during sex or an increase in the frequency of urinary-tract infections. Age-related pelvic-support disorders – such as the weakening of the muscles, connective tissue, and ligaments that hold the uterus and vagina in place – may also interfere with participation in and enjoyment of sex.

For men, the physical changes (to penis, scrotum, testicles, and prostate gland) are gradual. They tend to show up most noticeably in the penis. At age 40, about 25 percent of men fail to achieve an erection at least half the time; by age 70, it jumps to 52 percent; by age 80, it's over 75 percent. There are a number of common changes.

■ Sperm production in the testes declines, decreasing the amount of sperm available for ejaculation as well as the production of hormones, especially testosterone, necessary to stimulate interest in sex.

■ The sex drive (libido) decreases, often resulting in psychological (or performance) anxiety.

■ Blood flow to the spongy tissue of the penis decreases and/or slows, making it more difficult to obtain an erection without outside stimulation.

■ Erections do not remain firm enough for penetration or are lost before orgasm.

■ Orgasm does not always result in ejaculation, and/or the ejaculate is forced back up the penis into the bladder (retrograde ejaculation).

■ The time it takes to have another erection increases, in some cases up to twenty-four to forty-eight hours.

■ In addition, changes affecting the prostate often lead to bladder control problems, urinary-tract infections, or prostate cancer.

It's not just about the equipment

The physical changes taking place below the belly button are just one of the factors that can play havoc with the ability to have an intimate and fulfilling sex life as you age.

Drugs That May Cause Erectile Dysfunction in Men

Anticonvulsants

Anti-infective drugs

Cardiovascular drugs
  Antiarrhythmics
  Antihypertensives
    Adrenergic blockers (centrally or
    peripherally acting)
    ß-Blockers
    Calcium channel blockers
    Clonidine
    Direct vasodilators
    Diuretics
    Reserpine

Drugs affecting the CNS
  Alcohol
  Anxiolytics and sedative-hypnotics
  Antidepressants
  Antipsychotics
  CNS stimulants
  Cocaine

Drugs affecting the CNS (continued)
  Levodopa
  Lithium
  Narcotics

Gastrointestinal drugs
  Anticholinergics and antispasmodics
  H_2 blockers
  Metoclopramide

Miscellaneous drugs
  Acetazolamide
  Baclofen
  Cimetidine
  Clofibrate
  Danazol
  Disulfiram
  Estrogens
  Interferon
  Leuprolide
  Naproxen
  Progesterone

CNS = central nervous system.

Adapted from "Impotence," by T.H. Stanisic and G.E. Francisco, in *Geriatric Pharmacology*, edited by R. Bressler and M.D. Katz. New York, McGraw-Hill, 1993, p. 272. Used with permission.

The illnesses and chronic conditions you're dealing with, especially diabetes, heart disease, and depression, play a role, too. Diabetes, because of its effect on the arteries and capillaries, is a direct cause of erectile dysfunction, and it's probably a contributing factor to the loss of vaginal lubrication in women. Recent research has shown that problems with premature ejaculation that occur in a man's 40s or 50s may actually be an early warning sign of cardiovascular disease. The role depression has in throwing a wet blanket on intimacy and sexuality has been well documented. (*See Conditions and Illnesses That Affect Sexual Function, page 114.*)

The aftereffects of medical treatments (especially for cancer) and surgery play a role as well. Despite the fact that a mastectomy (removal of all or part of the breast), hysterectomy (removal of the uterus), or oophorectomy (removal of the ovaries) does not lessen or interfere with sexual desire, many women feel "less feminine" after surgery. A prostatectomy (removal of the prostate) may cause total loss of penis function and/or urinary incontinence.

Both prescription and over-the-counter medications can play havoc with libido and performance. Worst offenders include antihistamines, antidepressants, antipsychotics, tranquilizers, appetite suppressants, ulcer medications, and medications prescribed for hypertension and diabetes. (*See Drugs That May Cause Erectile Dysfunction, page 110,* and *Possible Effects of Drugs on Female Sexuality, page 113.*)

Alcohol can put the kibosh on intimacy, too, especially for older adults. One drink, especially if it's part of a romantic dinner, can act as an aphrodisiac by stimulating desire, increasing relaxation, and lowering inhibitions. Heavy drinking, however, dulls the senses and "relaxes" things so much that men can't achieve an erection and women can't achieve an orgasm.

And finally, what's going on in your head plays a role in intimacy and sexuality that's equal in importance to what's going on with all the physical parts. Even if all the equipment is in A-1 working order, if one partner is worried about performing or the other partner is worried about a recent fender-bender or the loss of a friend, little or nothing is going to happen between the two. If both parties aren't focused on the moment, that lack of focus has an immediate and direct effect on what they'll be able to respond to, experience, and enjoy.

And, speaking of enjoyment, when you read all those books and listen to all those talk shows about sexuality and intimacy, if you think they're only talking about intercourse, you have blinders on. Sexuality has different meanings for different people, and the older you get the broader the definition of the word becomes.

Sex and the Senior Set: Myth #3

Myth: *Older adults are not attractive and therefore not sexually desirable.*

Reality: Ideals about what constitutes beauty and handsomeness are in the eye of the beholder. And they change over time, becoming spiced, seasoned, and nuanced with the experience, wisdom, and insight that come with bifocals, graying hair, and the ability to see further than skin-deep.

Sex and the Senior Set: Myth #4

Myth: *Older adults don't need to practice safe sex.*

Reality: Sexually transmitted diseases (STDs) are equal-opportunity ogres. Not only has the incidence of STDs like chlamydia, herpes, and genital warts (human papillomavirus) increased in the over-60 population, but so has the incidence of AIDS.

At 21, enthusiastic and athletic coupling may be what intimacy is all about. However, as you age sexual expression evolves into a broad range of physical and emotional acts. For some, sexuality is the sharing of warmth, tenderness, and emotional intimacy; for others, it's companionship; some associate it with touching and being touched. For most, however, it's the conscious weaving together of intercourse and the vast array of "outercourse" options (hand-holding, kissing, cuddling, whole-body massage, oral sex, sharing of fantasies, etc.) that provide the stimulation, pleasure, intimacy, fulfillment, and life-affirming connectedness that are the hallmarks of a sexual relationship that's physically and emotionally satisfying, whether you're 21 or 101.

Taking care of business

Adding years means adding activities to the romance repertoire, not subtracting them.

If you're experiencing the low libido and intermittent or chronic sexual dysfunction that can come with aging, you should seek help for the problem. In most cases, your physician can diagnose the problem with a thorough medical history, physical exam, and blood and urine tests, and prescribe treatment. However, in cases where the problem may be a secondary symptom of a chronic or medically complex condition, referral to a urologist, gynecologist, or endocrinologist may be necessary.

Mars: It's a guy thing

The most common problems men face are premature ejaculation, erectile dysfunction, and low libido. Men dealing with diminished libido, reduced sensitivity to sexual stimulation, decreased orgasm intensity, and the depression that can often accompany these symptoms may be suffering from hypogonadism (low levels of the male hormone testosterone) and may benefit from testosterone therapy. It can be administered as a gel, patch, or biweekly injection, and has been shown to improve not only libido, but also muscle strength, mood, and sense of overall well-being.

The treatment for premature ejaculation and erectile dysfunction has changed dramatically since the introduction of Viagra, Cialis, and Levitra, all of which increase blood flow to the penis. Today, 70 percent of erectile-dysfunction patients are leaving their physician's office with a prescription for one of these pills. Those who can't use these drugs, such as those taking nitroglycerin to treat heart disorders, can get the same effect through the use of injections or pellets inserted into the penis. In addition, mechanical devices such as penis rings, vacuum pumps, and surgically implanted pumps are available.

Possible Effects of Drugs on Female Sexuality

Effect	Drug
Increased sexual desire	Androgens, benzodiazepines (antianxiety effect), mazindol
Decreased sexual desire	Some of the drugs that decrease libido in men may reduce libido in women. The literature on this subject is sparse.
Impaired arousal and orgasm	Anticholinergics, clonidine, methyldopa, monoamine, oxidase inhibitors, selective serotonin reuptake inhibitors, tricyclic antidepressants
Breast enlargement	Estrogens, penicillamine, tricyclic antidepressants
Galactorrhea (spontaneous flow of milk)	Amphetamines, chlorpromazine, cimetidine, haloperidol, heroin, methyldopa, metoclopramide, phenothiazine, reserpine, sulpiride, tricyclic antidepressants
Virilization (acne, hirsutism, lowered voice, clitoral enlargement)	Androgens, haloperidol

Adapted from "Many common medications can affect sexual expression," by J.W. Long, *Generations* 6:32-34. Reprinted with permission from *Generations, Journal of the American Society on Aging*, 833 Market Street, Suite 512, San Francisco, California 94103. Copyright 1981, ASA.

Conditions and Illnesses That Affect Sexual Function

Alcoholism	High cholesterol levels
Anxiety (including performance anxiety)	Hypertension (high blood pressure)
	Hypogonadism
Arthritis	(low hormone levels)
Cancer	Hypotension (low blood pressure)
Cerebrovascular disease	Kidney disease
Coronary artery disease	Liver disease
Chronic-fatigue syndrome	Obesity
Chronic obstructive pulmonary disease (COPD)	Parkinson's disease
	Peripheral vascular disease
Chronic pain	Pituitary disease
(especially of the back)	Pulmonary and lung disease
Depression	Substance abuse
Diabetes	(of both alcohol and illegal drugs)
Fibromyalgia	Thyroid disease

Venus: Quality time

Women who are dealing with decreased libido can often improve sexual response by working with their partners to add more tactile "spice" – foreplay, cuddling, massage – to their lovemaking, because for many women the skin often acts as the body's largest sex organ. Or they may be candidates for estrogen or testosterone therapy, both of which decrease after menopause. While it's not for every woman, studies indicate that testosterone therapy can increase libido and pleasure for many women, including those who have undergone hysterectomies.

Those who are dealing with painful intercourse resulting from a decrease in vaginal lubrication and the thinning of the vaginal walls are candidates for vaginal lubricants and moisturizers, and may also be candidates for localized estrogen therapy. (*See Sex Enhancers for Women, page 118.*)

Those who are dealing with urine leakage during sex (stress incontinence), which can make the experience both uncomfortable and embarrassing, are candidates for nonsurgical treatment with Kegel exercises or the insertion of a vaginal pessary. Kegels strengthen the pelvic floor and the muscles supporting the vagina; a pessary is a tiny silicone, plastic, or rubber device that supports the vagina so that it does not put pressure on the bladder.

When the going gets bumpy

You can probably chalk up about 90 percent of the intimacy problems couples have as they age to the physical changes that come with aging as well as to the chronic conditions related to aging and the medications used to treat them. Psychological factors account for the remaining 10 percent, and those problems can often be difficult to remedy.

For most people, the road to a satisfying sex life in their later years is paved throughout their relationship with the same negotiating and compromising that comes with being in a long-term relationship. However, there are times when sexual counseling or therapy may be needed to right the relationship. For example, if there has always been a wide difference between the partners' levels of desire and sexual interest, if the relationship has taken a severe physical or emotional hit through illness or an affair, or if the disparity in sexual interest has reached the point where one partner feels pressured and resentful while the other feels unloved, deprived, and desperate, counseling may be the answer.

The sooner the couple addresses the problem, the better. That's because treatment for the depression and other emotional issues (feelings of disappointment, guilt, stress, anger, etc.) that often come with disparities in sexual desire usually requires a coordinated plan that includes talk therapy, behavior modification strategies, and/or medications that may be used to treat both psychological and sexual dysfunction. Social workers, marriage counselors, and psychologists are usually able to work with people who have mild to moderate relationship problems. For those with severe problems or who are dealing with long-standing issues, however, it's best to seek counseling from a psychiatrist who is licensed to prescribe medications.

Counseling can definitely be a win-win situation that enriches both the sexual and emotional sides of a relationship. But it only works when both partners are willing to participate. If one is sitting in the therapist's office just to say "I gave it my best shot," both are wasting their time.

Their next move may be into separate bedrooms … or a lawyer's office.

Andropause: The ADAM Syndrome

Women go through menopause in their 50s. While men don't go through the sudden drop in hormones that is the hallmark of menopause, they do begin to experience a diminishing level of testosterone production in the testes (gonads) around that time. Called the ADAM (Androgen Deficiency in the Aging Male) syndrome, andropause, viropause, or male menopause, this drop in testosterone causes decreased libido with accompanying sexual dysfunction as well as decreased muscle strength, memory lapses, diminished energy, and depression. Those dealing with a severe case of ADAM syndrome also may have an increase in insomnia and appetite, along with anxiety and mood swings.

The good news about ADAM is that, when there are no underlying complications, it can usually be treated with injections, patches, or gels that boost the bioavailability of testosterone in the blood.

Testosterone is linked to prostate cancer, and taking supplements raises the level of the prostate-cancer marker PSA (prostate-specific antigen) in the blood. So those who are taking the supplement must be carefully monitored by their physician.

Counseling 101: Sex ed for silver foxes

Whether you're 60, 70, or 80, you are probably interested in maintaining a vital, intimate, and satisfying sex life. If you're experiencing a bit of trouble adjusting to the age-related physical changes that come with being a silver fox, or your partner is, one or more of the following strategies may be just what the doctor ordered.

- Talk to your partner, and make sure it's in a neutral space, not the bedroom. Being open and communicative about what is and isn't working and what is and isn't pleasurable soothes anxiety, boosts libido, and enhances "performance."

- Avoid initiating sex at times of the day when pain, fatigue, or stress levels are high. For many people, morning sex is best. In the morning, both partners are well rested, and older men are more likely to have an erection then.

- Focus on foreplay. Aging causes a decrease in the flow of blood to both male and female genitals. Increasing genital stimulation increases blood flow, which increases sexual desire and fulfillment for both men and women.

- Expand your sexual repertoire. When you think about sex, don't limit activity to the bedroom. Don't limit it to one or two tried-and-true positions either. Anything that becomes routine can lose its appeal over time. Be imaginative. There's a vast array of fulfilling activities beyond the basics. Give any or all of these a try: cuddling, kissing, showering together, massage, mutual masturbation, erotic literature, oral sex, and shared fantasies. One of these may turn out to be just what the doctor ordered.

- Get help. How-to books, pain medications, penis rings, "the little blue pill," lubricants and moisturizers, and sex toys are a win-win when it comes to sex. They lower performance anxiety and increase endurance and pleasure, too.

- Limit alcohol and tobacco use. Both constrict the blood vessels feeding the genitals.

- Get physical. You can't expect to perform in the bedroom if the other twenty-three hours of the day you're not giving your heart, lungs, and muscles a good workout.

Sex Enhancers for Women

Whether you're 55 or 75, vaginal dryness can turn a stimulating and pleasurable act into a tedious and painful encounter. It doesn't have to be that way if you come prepared.

Vaginal lubricants decrease friction during intercourse and add to pleasure. For health reasons, water-soluble lubricants such as Astroglide, Moist Again, Lubrin, and K-Y Personal Lubricant are highly recommended by the North American Menopause Society (NAMS), a group that's made it its business to know what women want.

NAMS says that oil-based lubricants don't make the cut at all. They're vehicles for infections.

Water-based vaginal moisturizers, such as Replens and K-Y Long Lasting Vaginal Moisturizer, are highly recommended. Because they act directly on tissue to decrease dryness and also contain elements that help maintain the vagina's acidic environment, they may be the best option for women who are prone to vaginal infections or who have symptoms of vaginal irritation or burning during intercourse.

In extreme cases, NAMS suggests short-duration use of local estrogen therapy, such as Premarin Vaginal Cream, Estrace Vaginal Cream, or the Estring Vaginal Ring. The latter is so mild that it is used by women undergoing cancer treatment.

Supplements and creams marketed for sexual "enhancement" get a solid thumbs-down rating from NAMS. If you choose to use them anyway, be aware that most contain ingredients such as "natural" oils, vitamin E, L-arginine, licorice extract, and black cohosh, which could interact with medications (especially blood thinners). So see your physician before using them.

Chapter 9
Working the System
So the System Works for You

When 79-year-old Jean B. called about coming in for a talk on knee replacement surgery, I wasn't surprised. She'd been complaining about both her knees for a couple of years, and the last time she came in seeking stronger pain medication, I suggested knee-replacement surgery.

She had laughed dismissively. "Surgery's not something a woman my age wants to talk about," she said.

Now she was ready to talk. But before the conversation could start, she needed to get a full set of knee x-rays so that she and I could see what and where the problems were. She also needed to come in for a blood workup and a full physical. Surgery is risky at any age, but when you have high blood pressure and osteoarthritis as Jean did, the risk goes up.

Jean got lucky. The nurse was able to schedule her x-rays and lab work for the same day, so we scheduled her physical and consult for a week later.

When she came in for her appointment, she was using a cane. When I asked her when that had started, she rolled her eyes and said, "It's been a couple of months now. It makes me feel old."

The orthopedic surgeon's report on Jean's x-rays recommended surgery on both knees done three months apart. Her lab report was good – though her lipids were higher than I'd have liked – and I gave her a clean bill of health on her physical.

Since there was no hurry for Jean's surgery, we talked about the best time to schedule both surgeries and what she expected them to accomplish. Because Jean had worked in health care for more than thirty years, her expectations were realistic. During an extended office visit, we put together a hospitalization, surgery, and discharge plan that included a patient-specific after-care and rehabilitation strategy.

Plan in hand, Jean went home, and she and her husband spent the next month getting ready for surgery. They cooked meals and stored them in the freezer. They stocked the medicine cabinet with surgical dressings and

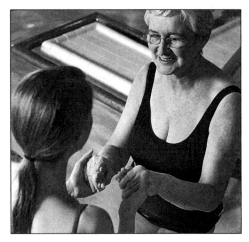

ointments. They went out and bought a walker and side-arm chair. "So I could push myself up with its arms," she explained.

Jean called the rehabilitation therapist I'd suggested and scheduled twelve weeks of rehab. And, because we'd discussed the fact that the more physically fit she was when she went into surgery, the faster and better she'd heal, she gave up her after-dinner cigarette and set up an exercise area complete with ankle weights and muscle-strengthening TheraBands in her den at home to strengthen the muscles in her thighs and calves.

Jean's surgery went so well that the surgeon asked her whether she'd mind his bringing a couple of surgical fellows in to see her, and her pre-op prep paid off handsomely. While she had planned to go to a nursing home for post-hospital care, the day before she was scheduled to be discharged she decided against it. Despite that decision, which I did not agree with, her knee wounds healed well, and she sailed through both six-week stints of physical therapy three days per week.

In fact, when Jean had the second knee replaced and the therapist called to give me a progress update, he was singing her praises. "Usually people her age come in and you have to push and push. With her, it's 'What else can I do?' 'Shouldn't I be on the treadmill longer?' 'Shouldn't I be using a heavier weight for leg lifts?' I wish everyone you sent me was like her."

So do I.

Health baggage

"Advanced age" is a catch phrase for the health baggage you collect over time. You're carrying it when you go into a hospital, make an office visit to consult with a physician, have a procedure done at an outpatient clinic, undergo physical therapy at a rehabilitation center, are discharged to a skilled-nursing facility to recover from an illness, or go into a nursing home for long-term care after a stroke.

Baggage is a hoary mix of:

■ **Genes**. The diseases, conditions, and physical impairments to which you are heir.

■ **Environment**. What you're exposed to that puts you in harm's way, such as viruses, germs, and situations.

■ **Lifestyle habits**. What you do or don't do through the years to keep your lungs free of cancer, your weight under control, your cardiovascular system tuned up, etc.

■ **Health-maintenance habits**. Preventive maintenance, such as checkups, screenings, vaccinations, yearly physicals, medical procedures, and treatments that you do or don't pursue as you age to keep your body tuned up and chronic diseases at bay.

■ **The multiplier effect**. The combined impact on your physical and health status of the injuries, illnesses, diseases, and chronic conditions that you have accumulated over time.

As you age, the influence each of these bits of baggage has on your current and future health alters. When you're young, genes and environment play a major role in what you will and won't come down with and how well your body will deal with each situation. As you get older, building on what genes and environment have laid down, lifestyle and health-maintenance habits move to the fore in shaping your health status. By the time you hit late middle age, the conditions that have accumulated over time take over as the major predictor and manifestation of health status.

Surveys indicate that by age 65, 30 percent of people have at least one chronic condition that is serious enough to require medications or medical treatment, or both. The most common are diabetes, heart disease, high blood pressure, arthritis, and cancer.

But, as I explained in Chapter 2, one chronic condition can trigger the development of a cluster of conditions and illnesses as you age. For instance, uncontrolled high blood pressure opens the door to cerebrovascular disease, which opens the door to strokes, which opens the door to dementia. Unmanaged diabetes opens the door to cardiovascular disease, which opens the door to heart disease and blindness due to diabetic retinopathy.

But the interplay of chronic conditions isn't the only factor affecting your health status and your ability to fight off diseases as you age. Age-related wear and tear take their toll on joints, muscles, and tissue. And the ability of the immune system to fight off diseases and germs and promote recovery after an illness or injury declines. At some point on the aging arc, the physical reserves (called homeostatic reserves) needed to successfully maintain your health and recover after a "hit," whether it's a broken finger or a heart attack, begin to decline. Initially, it's a gradual decline. You notice that it takes longer for a cut to heal or longer to get over a cold. But as the years and the baggage pile up, the decline speeds up.

It's a rare individual who reaches the 70s or 80s without having diseases and conditions that make dealing with the health-care system risky business. And, as people push into their 80s, the cognitive decline that comes with reaching very old age (50 percent of those 85 and over have some form of dementia) is added to the baggage.

The flip side of this seemingly bad news is that preventive behaviors like eating smart, exercising, and getting your physicals, tests, and vaccinations, pay huge health dividends as you age. And it's never too late to start taking care of yourself.

Vigilance also pays off. You can heed what your body is telling you by recognizing the situations, transition periods, and signs that herald changes in your health status and physical function. If you subsequently address them by modifying your lifestyle and increasing your health-maintenance activities, you can head into old age in optimal condition – in such optimal condition, in fact, that your encounters with the health-care system will usually result in what doctors call "good outcomes."

But you can't do it alone.

What is a geriatrician?

Geriatricians are subspecialists in a field that's been around only since 1979. All complete three-year residencies in internal medicine or family practice medicine. Then they do an additional year of training (called a fellowship) in geriatric medicine, focusing on the syndromes, conditions, illnesses, and diseases that are unique to old age (macular degeneration, Alzheimer's disease, heart failure) or that are very common in old age (high blood pressure, diabetes, arthritis). In addition, they get hands-on experience in everything from geriatric wound care to cardiac rehabilitation to the diagnosis and treatment of the psychological and emotional issues of older adults.

The training is complex because geriatricians treat people with complex and interacting medical conditions such as arthritis, heart disease, depression, diabetes, kidney failure, and Alzheimer's disease.

By necessity, geriatricians are team players. Their teams include other medical specialists, nurses, pharmacists, social workers, rehabilitation specialists, social-service agencies, and family members. Some subspecialize, becoming geriatric neurologists or geriatric psychiatrists

Recent studies have shown that older patients who receive geriatric care tend to experience less physical decline, better mental health, and fewer moves to long-term-care facilities. But just because you hit 70 or 75 doesn't mean you should be seeing a geriatrician. There's no health advantage to seeing a geriatrician if you're well.

Indications that you may need to seek geriatric care include:

- Need for treatment of a specific condition, such as incontinence or debilitating osteoarthritis
- Inability to carry out the normal activities of daily living, such as bathing, taking care of the home, paying bills
- Dealing with two or three potentially life-threatening diseases and/or multiple chronic diseases
- Inability to follow a medical treatment plan and/or medication regimen that may include taking dozens of pills a day
- Confusion, memory loss, or periodic blackouts
- Loss of enjoyment of previously pleasurable activities
- Malnutrition resulting in noticeable weight loss
- Feelings of isolation, depression, listlessness
- Frequent falls resulting in bruises or broken bones
- Loss of bladder control
- Repeated 911 calls, emergency room visits, and/or hospital admissions
- Significant caregiver and/or family stress due to care of and worries about an elderly loved one

These triggers tend to appear around the time people turn 75 and/or during significant health or emotionally stressful transitions, such as the loss of a spouse, diagnosis of a second or third major disease, a stroke, or a fall that results in partial disability.

How to find a geriatrician

Among almost 660,000 physicians in the United States, fewer than 9,000 are geriatricians.

The best place to begin a search for a geriatrician is with your primary care physician. Another good source of referrals is agencies that deal with aging issues, such as adult day-care centers, social-service agencies, and disease-specific agencies, such as the Alzheimer's Association or Arthritis Foundation. Word of mouth is also a good source for referrals. But not everyone with a lot of older patients is a geriatrician. Geriatricians are board-certified. When you call a physician's office, ask whether the physician has a Certificate of Added Qualification (CAQ).

Getting a name is the first step in finding a geriatrician. The second step is a face-to-face meeting in which you ask lots of questions, including:

- Why did you go into geriatrics?
- Where and when did you get your geriatric training?
- Where do you have hospital privileges?
- How much time will you spend with me?

The oil that makes the wheels of the patient-physician relationship turn smoothly is time, which means that the physician can listen and work with each patient in order to arrive at medical decisions that incorporate understanding of and respect for the patient's wishes and values.

Partners in health

Whether you're 25 or 50 or 75, if you want to stay healthy you need to team up with a primary care physician or PCP. Think of a PCP as not only your health gatekeeper but also your partner in health. PCPs are on call when health problems and emergencies come up. They keep you healthy by scheduling and coordinating the physical exams, screens, and lab tests that catch symptoms before they become problems. They coordinate the services, procedures, and care you'll need to regain your health and function if you're hit with an injury, disease, or condition that requires outpatient treatment, surgery, hospitalization, or rehabilitation. And they offer a knowledgeable shoulder to cry on.

If you don't already have a primary care physician or are not satisfied with the one that you're currently seeing, call the best hospital in your area, or ask friends or co-workers for recommendations. You also can call your city's medical association or physician-referral service, or the state medical association. If you live near a medical school or university-based medical center, call its physician-referral service.

Shopping for a Primary Care Physician

Shopping for a primary care physician can be time-consuming, but the time spent ensuring the right "fit" will pay big dividends down the line.

Get a list of names and phone numbers of physicians from family, friends, acquaintances working in the health-care field, or physician organizations. If a doctor's name comes up more than once, put a star by it.

Then interview each doctor on the list to find out:

- The age and type of patients making up the majority of the practice
- Where the doctor was educated and served his/her residency and fellowship
- How long the doctor has been in practice
- Whether the doctor is board-certified or qualified in an area or specialty
- The doctor's communication style, philosophy, and approach to patient care, treatment, and management
- Location, accessibility, and office hours (especially during evenings and weekends)
- Where the doctor sends lab work and his/her affiliation with the lab
- Which hospitals and skilled nursing facilities the doctor sends patients to
- Who covers for the doctor in an emergency
- The type of health insurance the doctor accepts
- Whether the doctor has been involved in any lawsuits

The older you are, the more important it is to partner with a primary care physician. That doesn't mean that your age should be the major criterion for choosing him or her. The number of chronic conditions you're dealing with, the degree of care you require, and the doctor's access to the best hospital in your area (and to people with the expertise your doctor doesn't have) should carry the most weight. So, depending on that criterion, you could partner with a family practice physician, an internist, or a geriatrician.

Family practice physicians are the Dr. Welbys of today's medicine. They provide comprehensive care for people from birth through old age and are a good choice for healthy older people and those dealing with the most common conditions of aging, such as arthritis, osteoporosis, or high blood pressure.

Internists – sometimes called adult-medicine specialists – care for and treat the diseases and conditions affecting adults. Many specialize, becoming cardiologists, nephrologists, neurologists, oncologists, etc.

When a Geriatric Assessment Can Help

A geriatric assessment is usually warranted if an elderly patient has a severe chronic condition such as cancer or heart disease and two or more of the following:

- Multiple health problems
- Confusion or memory loss
- Behavioral changes (including depression)
- Difficulty performing daily activities
- Physical weakness, frailty
- Extreme weight loss or malnutrition
- Difficulty swallowing or breathing
- Difficulty managing multiple medications
- Difficulty walking or balancing
- Loss of bladder or bowel control
- Osteoarthritis or osteoporosis
- Significant functional decline (including falls)

An assessment usually requires more than one session and has four purposes. It empowers patients and their families to make informed health-care decisions; it helps shape a care plan and treatment goals that will best serve the patient; it identifies problems related to the person's cognitive, physical, and functional status that may interfere with mobility, independence, and quality of life; and it links patients and families with resources, such as support groups and community services, that will best serve their needs.

Following an assessment, a geriatrician explains its findings and provides patient and family with a written report and recommendations.

Geriatricians are the only physicians who are certified in the care of the elderly. Using a holistic model of care that focuses on patients' social and emotional needs as well as their health-care requirements, they assess, diagnose, treat, and coordinate the care of older adults with complex medical problems.

It's difficult to pinpoint exactly who should partner with a geriatrician. Because people in their 60s, 70s, and 80s are carrying so much baggage, their health-care needs are more specialized than those of people in their 30s, 40s, and 50s. However, in general, those who are going to derive the most benefit from partnering with a geriatrician are people in their 80s who are making a transition to a lower level of function and a greater level of dependence. This includes those experiencing physical or cognitive changes; those dealing with chronic conditions that require multiple medications, careful management, and coordinated care; those who are frail and prone to falling; and/or those who require a geriatric assessment to help them and their family members plan for the future.

Most older adults are going to be well cared for by family-practice physicians or internists because 95 percent of the people walking into their offices will be coming in with the typical diseases and conditions that accompany aging. When they encounter a situation that is so complex – for instance, a bladder infection on top of the patient's badly managed diabetes and high blood pressure – that it requires a second set of eyes and ears, they consult with a specialist.

The Education of a Geriatrician

To become a geriatrician, a physician must complete four years of medical school and a three-year residency in either family practice or internal medicine, and then serve a one-year fellowship in geriatric medicine at an academic-medical facility that has a department of geriatrics. In 2006, the year hundreds of thousands of baby boomers began turning 60, there were 370 physicians in geriatric fellowships. When physicians complete the fellowship and every ten years thereafter, they must pass a certificate-of-added-qualification (CAQ) exam. Then they can call themselves geriatricians.

Getting Ready for Surgery

Often you can't plan in advance for a trip to the hospital, but if you're going in for a scheduled or elective procedure, the fitter you are going in, the more quickly you'll recover and get out.

If you're carrying extra pounds, drop them. They slow recovery by putting a strain on the heart and circulatory system. And fat – adipose tissue on the operating table – interferes with surgical procedures and wound healing, which can lead to infections.

If you're underweight, add weight with nutrition supplements, such as Boost or Ensure, and, if you're up to it, an exercise program that builds muscle mass. Taking extra muscle mass to the hospital with you means that you'll have protein and glycogen reserves available for healing. If you're going in for joint surgery, get your physician's permission to do exercises that tone, strengthen, and stimulate the tissue, bone, and muscle around the joint being operated on.

Consult with your physician about the vitamin and mineral supplements you might be able to take to boost healing and recovery.

Cut out tobacco, caffeine, and alcohol, or you may suffer withdrawal symptoms during recovery. And tobacco interferes with circulation, so it slows healing.

If the patient is 60, the internist will probably consult a urologist. At 80, however, the patient probably will be referred to a geriatrician.

Because geriatricians deal with complicated and emotional cases, they head up teams that always include geriatric nurse specialists, case managers, and social workers. In addition, depending on whether the geriatrician is in an urban or rural area and operating out of a hospital or office, the team may also include psychiatrists or psychologists, pharmacists, occupational and physical therapists, dietitians, speech therapists, podiatrists, and "on-call" specialists in everything from urology to neurology.

When you're caring for people with the complicated, interacting, and often long-standing conditions that many older people bring into the geriatrician's office, being able to call upon a specialist is a necessity. Specialists have the expertise to perform the appropriate lab tests and work-ups needed to make

Deposit a couple of pints of your blood (an autologous donation) in the hospital's blood bank. If there is an emergency, with your blood on hand, there's no chance of a mismatch. If it's not used, donate it to the hospital.

Get yourself in better psychological shape as well. Get educated about the procedure you're having done, how long recovery will take and what it will entail, and, if you'll be going into rehab, what you can expect there. To do that:

- Get a second opinion.

- Get as much information as possible on the procedure you're undergoing from sources such as the surgeon, books, videos, others who have undergone the procedure, and the National Institutes of Health's health topics site: www.nlm.nih.gov/medlineplus/health topics.html.

- Discuss your feelings and fears with your doctor, family members, a hospital social worker, and/or a spiritual adviser.

- Meet with the rehabilitation team so that you understand what rehab is (and isn't) and to get a realistic time frame for recovery.

- Sign up for yoga or meditation classes, and learn stress-reduction and pain-management skills that you can take to the hospital with you.

- Get your personal affairs in order, just in case.

definitive diagnoses, sort out and prioritize symptoms and treatment options, and help manage the patient's treatment and follow-up care or hospitalization.

Going to the hospital

Hospitals are for acute situations, not smoldering chronic ones. You don't want to go to the hospital unless it's the absolute, no-doubt-about-it best place for you.

Hospitals are noisy. They're teeming with bacteria, germs, and viruses. They're rigidly run. They have "adverse incident" rates, which is medicalese for everything from staff dispensing the wrong medication to urinary-tract infections resulting from clogged catheters and bedsores resulting from prolonged bed rest, all of which keeps malpractice lawyers in business. They're staffed by extremely dedicated and incredibly overworked employees.

Hospitals are for those who have undergone surgical procedures that require post-surgical care or who are recovering from traumatic accidents or receiving treatment for acute illnesses and conditions.

If you can have your surgery done in an outpatient clinic or surgery center, don't go to a hospital.

If you have a nonacute illness such as a festering wound, low-grade pneumonia, or an infection that can be treated in the doctor's office and then managed at home, don't go.

If your doctor wants to send you to the hospital "just to run some tests and sort things out," don't go.

If your family wants to have you admitted to the hospital so that they can take a break from caregiving, don't go.

If your treatment and care are focused on comfort care and the palliation or control of pain, both of which you can receive as an outpatient or at home, don't go.

If you have a terminal illness but are comfortable with the idea of hospice care that will enable you to die at home in familiar circumstances, surrounded by family, don't go.

In other words, whether you're 40 or 60 or 80, don't go to the hospital unless it's not just one option but the *best* option for you.

If, on the other hand, you have an injury, attack, illness, or a worsening chronic condition that calls for you to be admitted to a hospital, choose your hospital carefully. And get there as quickly as possible. All the studies indicate that whether it's getting a bone set or receiving clot-busters for a stroke or antibiotics for a systemic infection, the more quickly treatment starts, the better the outcome in terms of both health and function.

If you're 70 or older, and the hospital has an Acute Care of the Elderly (ACE) unit, demand to be admitted to that floor. ACE unit nurses are specially trained in geriatrics and the use of minimally invasive therapies, and rooms are designed to address the unique needs of patients who may be frail, incontinent, and/or cognitively impaired.

Making sure you choose the best hospital for you is a critical step. Think about it. If you go to the best hospital in the area, you get the best care; if you go to the worst, you get adequate care at best. When you're hospitalized, whether for an elective procedure or an emergency, you don't want adequate care; you want the best-quality care possible.

Why, When, and How to Get a Second Opinion

Second opinions aren't for the average circumstances that show up in an office physical exam, lab test, or screening. They're for the tough calls, the situations where there's sufficient uncertainty regarding the accuracy of the diagnosis, the choice of a treatment option, or the patient's prognosis if one form of treatment is chosen over another. This is when it makes sense to run the exam, lab, and screening results by a second pair of expert eyes.

Where there's a tough call, it's always reasonable to request a second opinion. In fact, physicians who work in areas like cancer, cardiovascular disease, and dementia, where there are a lot of "gray areas," usually welcome a patient's request for a second opinion.

Some patients have their physician set up the consult. Others are more comfortable getting copies of exams and lab work and setting up consultations on their own. Both choices are appropriate.

Ironically, many older people are reluctant to seek a second opinion because they feel it will offend their physician. Patients are usually wrong about that, and if they're seeing a physician who doesn't suggest that they seek a second opinion or doesn't take their request for a second opinion seriously, they may want to think about getting another doctor, not just another opinion.

What are indicators that a hospital provides high-quality care?

One indicator is that the hospital attracts a high volume of patients with illnesses and conditions similar to yours. In medicine as in basketball, practice makes (almost) perfect. The more experience a hospital's surgeons, nursing staff, lab technicians, and rehab therapists have with patients who have undergone complicated procedures such as hip replacements, heart transplants, breast reconstructions, or spine fusions, the better they are at what they do.

A hospital that is affiliated with a university medical school is another good indicator. That means state-of-the art surgical strategies, medications, and therapies will be the norm; highly skilled specialists will be available for consults on a moment's notice; and ultra-high-tech equipment will be monitoring patient progress 24/7.

Choose a hospital with lab facilities that are open and staffed round the clock. Emergencies arise when they arise, not just from 9 a.m. to 5 p.m.

Look for a hospital with a nursing department that has been granted Magnet Status, an indicator of nursing excellence, by the American Nurses Association. While a doctor is the one who gets you admitted to a hospital and coordinates procedures and care, the floor nurses oversee patients' progress, monitor high-tech equipment, change dressings, and dispense medications, and they're the ones who are going to get you discharged.

See whether the hospital is ranked as a top pick by *U.S. News & World Report* or one of the hospital-ranking organizations. Just because a hospital isn't ranked doesn't mean that it's not good; it just means that it's not one of the top-ranked hospitals.

Check whether the hospital has a coordinated palliative-care program (sometimes called a comfort-care program) to alleviate the pain and suffering that often accompany a catastrophic or terminal illness.

Finally, find a hospital that provides a post-hospital care plan ensuring that upon discharge, whether home or to a skilled nursing facility, patients continue the recovery and rehabilitation that was begun in the hospital.

Where recovery really takes place

For most people, going to the hospital is step one on the journey back to health.

Step two is rehabilitation. In the hospital, treatment is given to make you better. Rehab is a whole other ballgame. If you aren't 100 percent involved in what's going on, progress is slow or nonexistent.

What you'll be doing in rehab and where you'll be doing it will depend on what brought you into the hospital, how you responded to what occurred there, and your discharge plan. People who know they'll be going into the hospital usually have a discharge plan in hand on the day they're admitted. Those who are brought in by ambulance usually have theirs in a couple of days. Whether created two days after admission or three weeks out, and regardless of where the patient is headed next, the discharge plan is the crucial road map back to function, vitality, and quality of life.

Plans are individualized and created by a team composed of the patient's hospital physician, the primary care physician, a nurse manager, a hospital-based social worker, family members or caregivers, and the patient.

On Death and Hospitals

People 65 and older make up only 13 percent of the U.S. population, yet they account for 36 percent of all hospitalizations and more than 80 percent of all the deaths that occur in hospitals. The easy explanation for those staggering hospitalization and death statistics is that more people over age 65 are going into hospitals today than at any other time in history, and the older you are when you're hit with a disease, condition, or "event" (heart attack, fall, car accident, etc.) that sends you into the hospital, the higher your probability of dying there. Advanced age is often listed on a death certificate as a major or contributing factor in a patient's death.

Physicians and nurses focus on the patient's medical needs and on educating patient and caregiver about them. If the patient is going home, they help the family locate supplies and equipment needed for recovery and outline the physical therapy programs and activities to be done at home or in a physical therapist's office. If the patient is going into a skilled-nursing facility, the discharge plan outlines the physical-therapy programs and activities that the patient should pursue in order to regain health, strength, and mobility. Never assume that the therapies, medications, and/or special equipment suggested in a discharge plan are covered by insurance or Medicare. Both *will* pay for them, but only when they're authorized by a physician as part of the patient's discharge plan.

To ensure that no problems arise, get everything in writing, and be sure to make copies.

The social worker focuses on the patient's and caregiver's emotional, psychological, and financial issues and helps locate social services such as transportation companies and support groups in the community. (*See Chapter 10 for more about caregiving.*)

When a discharge plan indicates that rehabilitation and/or recovery will take a long time or that rehabilitation will result in major lifestyle changes, contact support groups run by local organizations such as the Arthritis Foundation, American Heart Association, or American Cancer Society. Participants in these groups are dealing with similar situations. They can share insights and coping strategies that can help patients and caregivers regain a feeling of control.

When a cure isn't possible

Nobody goes to a hospital (or skilled-nursing facility or nursing home) to die, but no matter how dedicated doctors and nurses are and no matter how good hospitals are, sometimes the catastrophically ill or injured patients must go on life-support machines such as heart pumps, ventilators, and feeding tubes.

For many people, this is not an acceptable way to end their days. But unless they have taken the time to create advance directives and made sure that family members know about them *and* that the documents are in their patient file at the hospital or nursing home, that is what will happen.

An advance directive is a legal document that explains what type of care and support you want if you're no longer able to communicate your wishes while you're on life support.

A **living will** (also called a medical directive to doctors) is a written document that states what medical care, treatments, and medications you want and do not want.

A **do not resuscitate order** (DNR) is a directive to the attending physician and staff not to revive you if you go into cardiac arrest or your breathing stops.

A **health-care power of attorney** (HCPoA) is a document that gives a person (or persons) you designate the power to tell your care providers what you want in the event that you're not able to speak for yourself.

These documents are available free from most states' Department of Aging, the local Area Agency on Aging, hospitals, and most nursing homes. State-specific documents can be downloaded free from Caring Connections at www.caringinfo.org.

Getting a handle on hospice

Some people say that hospice means giving up. Some say that hospice shortens life or uses addictive drugs to treat patients.

Others say that hospice is about being in control and not having to deal with pain, and being able to be with family and loved ones all the way to the end.

Both are right.

While there are stand-alone hospices, and most hospitals have hospice beds or floors, hospice is not a *place*. It's a comprehensive program of comfort care, pain control, and psychological and social services that allow a terminally ill patient to manage pain, maintain quality of life, and remain at home. In fact, 80 percent of hospice services are delivered in the patient's home.

To receive hospice services, you must have six months or less to live, decide that you're no longer going to seek curative treatment, and "elect" to enroll in a program. Payment for the program is covered at a fixed daily rate by Medicare, Medicaid, and most private insurance.

Enrolling in a hospice program doesn't lock you into the program, however. If you're not satisfied with hospice's comfort-care model, you can opt back into a care-and-treatment program aimed at a cure.

Hospice care is team care. Members of the team include:

- The patient and designated family members
- The hospice's medical director, who draws up a care plan based on the patient's medical prognosis and goals
- A nurse, who sees the patient on a regular basis and is responsible for carrying out the care plan
- A social worker, who coordinates social services and offers supportive counseling
- A pharmacist, who dispenses pain medications
- Volunteers, who act as patient companions and provide respite for caregivers
- Home-health aides and technicians, who change dressings, set up medical equipment, collect test specimens, etc.
- Massage, physical, music, and art therapists.

All hospice care is palliative care, which is sometimes confusing. Palliative care is the use of prescription drugs to control pain. Hospice is more holistic. While it does use drugs to control pain, it also treats the mental, emotional, and spiritual needs of both patient and family members.

Chapter 10
Taking Care of the Caregiver

At 60, Doreen L. defines the phrase "sandwich generation." She's a full-time mother of a 13-year-old "bonus baby" and co-owner, with her husband, Howard, of a successful marketing business. And until recently, she was her 82-year-old widowed mother's sole caregiver.

Doreen says she can't remember when she took on that role. "It was when she started getting forgetful," she said. But she knows the exact moment when she realized that she had shed the helpful-daughter role and become a caregiver. "Five months ago, Mom had hip-replacement surgery, and as I was talking with the hospital discharge planner about where she'd go for rehab, she kept saying, 'As your mother's primary caregiver, you need to do this and you need to do that.'"

"That's when it dawned on me," said Doreen. "I *was* Mom's caregiver, and I'd been taking care of her for at least five years."

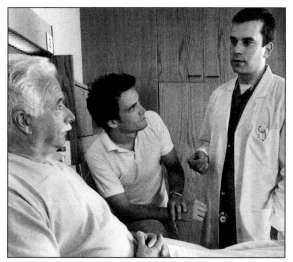

Other things dawned on her, too. Her need to spend four or five hours a day with her mother, as she'd been doing before her mother's surgery, was the reason she decided to start the business with her husband. "That way, I could work from home and have the flexibility I needed to take her shopping, do her laundry, tidy up the house, and get her to her doctor's appointments," Doreen explained.

It was the reason she'd allowed friendships to fall by the wayside. "People just stopped calling," she said. "One friend actually asked me if I was mad at her because I hadn't seen her in such a long time."

It was the reason she'd put on weight. "I was anxious and frustrated and nibbling all the time, and I quit going to the gym. Even though it's only about half a mile from the house, I just don't have time for it," she said.

It wasn't until her mother went into the skilled-nursing facility for rehab that Doreen met geriatric social worker Donna Mason, and her life became (more or less) her own again. "Donna hooked me up with a whole array of local services: adult day-care programs, home-companion services, meal-delivery programs, scheduled-transportation services, doctors who make house calls, online pharmacies that deliver prescription medications right to your doorstep," she said. "They haven't just lightened my caregiving responsibilities. They're also ensuring that Mom is maintaining her independence."

She added, "I just wish that Howard and I had known about all these services and programs five years ago."

The 80 Percent Quandary

About 80 percent of the family members I see come to me during a crisis.

Usually they're in crisis for one of two reasons. First, their spouse's or parent's mental and/or physical decline was so gradual that they didn't see a crisis-in-the-making, such as a fall that breaks a hip, a stove fire that burns the house down, an accident that totals the car and leaves the driver in a coma.

Or second, they did notice signs and symptoms, and might even have made an informed guess as to what they indicated, but they didn't want to interfere in an older person's life. Or they didn't want to deal with the family issues that would come up if someone actually said, "You know, Mom hasn't been herself. She's acting strangely. Maybe we ought to ask her what's going on or go to the doctor with her and have her checked out."

Instead, everyone walks around on eggshells. The crisis hits, and Mom ends up in the hospital or nursing home or…

Crossing the line

Like Doreen L., most people who have gradually assumed the role of primary caregiver don't see themselves as caregivers. It's not that they're in denial about what they're doing. They know that when they help their spouses find a word, sweater, or book, or they pick up their mothers-in-law every Saturday to go shopping, or they take their widowed aunts to doctors' appointments, they're helping. But they think they're simply being loving spouses, good sons, thoughtful nieces. This blinds them to the fact that they're providing essential care.

But at some point along the trajectory into caregiving, they cross the line that separates helping from caregiving and start turning into caregivers. Usually, this evolution is a slow, gradual, and anxiety-inducing process, as a spouse or parent or elderly relative becomes less active, more forgetful, and more frail.

Sometimes, however, they're thrust into the role of caregiver in a crisis, as when a 62-year-old husband has a massive stroke or an 82-year-old mother falls and breaks her hip. Both will come out of the hospital and rehab requiring far more time, energy, hands-on care, and emotional support than they did before their hospitalization. (*See Long-Distance Caregiving, page 149.*)

The stages of caregiving

Research indicates that there are seven recognizable stages in caregiving. Though the caregiving trajectory is the same for everyone, not everyone spends the same amount of time in each stage, and the lines of demarcation between the stages are fluid. Those who have good financial resources or a good support network at the time they assume the role of primary caregiver usually experience less emotional stress and physical strain during each stage.

Stage 1: This mainly consists of running the occasional errand and generally "being there" for spouse, parent, or friend. During this stage, caregivers are usually reacting to dropped hints ("I would so like to see that show downtown, but the traffic is so bad") or requests ("Since you pass right by the cleaners coming home from work, would you mind picking up my dry cleaning?"). Subconsciously, however, they may realize that they are providing care.

Stage 2: This is the point at which a caregiver recognizes the situation. He or she realizes that a significant amount of time and energy is being spent on things that may look and feel like just "being nice" or "being there," but are in reality activities that help the care recipient remain involved, independent, and healthy.

Stage 3: At this point, caregiver stress increases significantly. The caregiver must schedule significant blocks of time for caregiving activities and/or assume tasks involving personal care, such as feeding, bathing, or paying bills. This is usually the stage at which caregiving responsibilities begin conflicting significantly with family activities, home life, and since 59 percent of caregivers are employed, job responsibilities. This is often the stage at which many care recipients move in with or move closer to the caregiver.

Stage 4: This is the point at which the caregiver becomes so stressed that he or she begins seeking and using in-home services. Since increased caregiver burden and mild to moderate depression often go hand in hand, this is also the point at which many caregivers join support groups or seek psychological counseling. Having to coordinate and pay for all these services usually increases caregiver stress. (*See Help for Caregivers Is Just a Phone Call Away, page 144.*)

Stage 5: At this stage, care can no longer be safely provided or effectively coordinated by the primary caregiver, and the caregiver begins considering placement in a long-term-care facility or hospice program.

Stage 6: This is the stage at which placement is actually done.

Stage 7: At this stage, hands-on care decreases significantly as a result of placement in a nursing home or the death of the care recipient. While the physical strain of caregiving significantly decreases, grieving, feelings of guilt, and financial responsibilities during this stage may increase stress and depression levels for up to three years.

Dealing with depression

They're grieving the loss of a loved one. Their caregiving responsibilities leave them feeling isolated and lonely. They're angry – and feel guilty about the anger – at having to take on the role and responsibility of caregiver. They're juggling home and work and caregiving responsibilities. They may be caring for a mother, father, or sibling who doesn't realize that they're there or with whom they've never had an easy relationship. And they're depressed. Some are so emotionally numb that they don't realize they're depressed; others do, but deny it. Still others are self-medicating with alcohol or drugs.

Depression is a medical condition. It won't get better if it's not treated. Treatment depends on the severity of the depression. Mild to moderate depression can often be treated with psychotherapy or cognitive and behavioral therapy. Both help the caregiver identify and change negative, self-defeating thinking and behaviors. Moderate to severe depression may require "talk therapy" and prescription antidepressants such as Prozac, Zoloft, or Norpramin, which work on neurotransmitters in the brain. The medications help the mind become more receptive and responsive to the talk therapy.

Insurance and Medicare usually pay for some mental-health services. In addition, many companies' Employee Assistance Programs provide access to licensed therapists and/or psychologists, and many social-service agencies provide their services on a sliding fee scale.

The websites of the National Institute of Mental Health (www.nimh.nih. gov), National Association of Social Workers (www.naswdc.org), American Psychological Association (www.apa.org), and American Psychiatric Association (www.psych.org) provide good information on depression. The last three sites also provide information on how to find professionals in your area.

It's a Girl Thing #1

About a third of caregivers are spouses, primarily female. The other two-thirds are (in descending order) female adult children, daughters-in-law, male adult children, siblings, other relatives (e.g., grandchildren, nieces, nephews), female friends, and representatives of religious or social-work organizations.

The burden and blessing of caregiving

Whether they're 55-year-old daughters or 75-year-old husbands, if caregivers are trying to go it alone, they often experience early and intense emotional stress and physical strain, which lead to feelings of "caregiver burden" and physical and emotional burnout.

Feeling burdened and burned out has a negative effect on sleeping and eating patterns as well as on the immune system's ability to fight off germs and viruses. It also promotes the production of stress-related compounds, such as C-reactive protein (CRP) and interleukin-6, which increase the risk for and impact of many chronic conditions, such as cardiovascular disease, hypertension, diabetes, osteoporosis, and arthritis.

For caregivers who care for a spouse, burden and burnout can even have a terminal effect. According to a recent study, if you're a caregiving spouse, your risk of dying is 63 percent higher than it is for someone your age who is not a caregiver. According to another study that followed half a million couples, the caregiver's risk for an early death increases dramatically if the care recipient has had a stroke, hip fracture, or Alzheimer's disease and is hospitalized.

If caregiving sounds like a difficult and demanding undertaking, it is – particularly when the person you're caring for has a worsening chronic condition. Most of the caregivers who come into my office are devastated, not by what they're doing or what they're seeing, but by their feelings of helplessness and powerlessness as someone they love disappears before their eyes. Yet, they tell me, they wouldn't trade their time as a caregiver for anything.

Even when they have all the significant signs of caregiver stress and burnout, they tell me that what they are doing is "rewarding," "satisfying," "gratifying," and "fulfilling." And, when their caregiving comes to an end, they always say in one way or another, "I don't regret a moment of what I did."

Caregiver stress can lead to depression and burnout

Despite that fact that most caregivers ultimately see caregiving as rewarding, almost half of all caregivers become significantly depressed at some point in their caregiving career. Several interrelated factors contribute to how stressed, strained, burdened, and depressed you are as a caregiver. They include your gender and ethnic background, your relationship with the person you're caring for, the severity of that person's condition and needs, the location of your home and that of the care recipient, your financial resources and those of the care recipient, the support network available to you, and the duration of the caregiving situation.

While the perception of what is stressful and burdensome is different for each caregiving situation, the indicators of stress, emotional and physical overload, and depression are unerringly similar. Signs and symptoms include:

- Feelings of resentment, anger, impatience, and/or irritability at family members or the care recipient
- Guilt and inadequacy because you feel you aren't doing enough for the care recipient
- Anxiety because you feel inadequately informed yet overwhelmed with responsibilities
- Low energy, fatigue, and feelings of mental and physical exhaustion
- Feelings of apathy, including loss of libido and interest in once-pleasurable activities
- Feelings of sadness and spontaneous outbreaks of crying
- Mood swings
- Appetite changes that have led to weight loss or gain
- Insomnia or the inability to get out of bed in the morning
- Increased family stress resulting from family-caregiver conflicts
- Increased job stress resulting from job-caregiver conflicts
- Social isolation resulting from caregiving responsibilities that consume both time and money
- Increased "self-medication" with tobacco, alcohol, psychoactive medications, or illegal drugs
- Postponed or missed medical and dental appointments

Three or four of these symptoms indicate depression. Many caregivers exhibit many more than that.

It's a Girl Thing #2

Most women will spend seventeen years caring for children and eighteen years caring for a parent or elderly relative.

Help for Caregivers Is Just a Phone Call Away

The physical strain of caregiving – cooking, cleaning, lifting, bathing, dressing, driving to and from the doctor, etc. – and the emotional stress of trying to juggle family, job, and caregiver roles can be overwhelming. The following resources can help lighten the burden.

Care managers/care consultants/case managers: Care managers, most of whom charge by the hour, are usually specially trained nurses or social workers. They assess a care recipient's medical needs and home situation, then coordinate, schedule, manage and monitor care and services. They are especially valuable resources for those who are doing long-distance caregiving or caring for people with complex care needs. To locate a care manager, use the U.S. Administration on Aging's Eldercare Locator (www.eldercare.gov), or contact the National Association of Professional Geriatric Care Managers at 520-881-8008 or www.caremanager.org.

Local agencies and organizations: Your local Area Agency on Aging, Council on Aging, AARP group, United Way Agency, county Department of Family Services, religious organization (such as Catholic Charities or Jewish Family Services), or hospice can point you in the direction of services – Meals on Wheels, transportation, etc. These organizations will also be able to put you in touch with support groups and other programs that help caregivers recharge their batteries, meet others who are coping with similar situations and issues, and locate additional information and resources.

Taking care of number one

Of the things you should be doing as a caregiver, taking care of yourself is the most important and most often overlooked. If you end up weak and wobbly because you aren't eating right, you can't provide care. If you end up in the hospital with pneumonia because you're physically run-down, you can't provide care. If you end up so emotionally numb that you can't get out of bed in the morning, you can't provide care.

All this means that when you're a caregiver, you must step back and consciously identify the barriers to doing what it takes to stay physically strong and emotionally healthy. Then you must break those barriers down.

■ Recognize that you have added a new role – caregiver – to your life. When you spend a couple of hours a month returning your husband's books to

National organizations: Agencies and organizations dedicated to assisting people with chronic conditions and specific diseases, including the National Organization for Rare Diseases (www.rarediseases.org), are excellent sources for medical information and resources, caregiver information and coping strategies, and condition-specific specialists. Many can also provide information on the latest medical research and government-sponsored clinical trials.

Adult day care: These half- and full-day programs offer a place for older adults to socialize and engage in a variety of activities. Programs run on the Program of All-inclusive Care of the Elderly (PACE) model also provide medication, medical supervision, and other services.

Home health agencies: These nonprofit and for-profit agencies provide home health aides and registered nurses for short- or long-term care. The best way to locate a good agency is through hospital discharge planners and social workers or through word of mouth.

Nursing home or assisted-living facilities: When a respite is needed, both types of facilities may be able to provide short-term stays.

Employee Assistance Programs: If you're employed in a large company, you may be able to tap into caregiver resources through your company's human resources department or Employee Assistance Program.

the library, taking his clothes to the dry cleaner, and cleaning up after him in the kitchen, you're being nice. When you spend fifteen or twenty hours a week taking your mother shopping, straightening up her apartment, and doing her laundry, you're a caregiver. The sooner you can see a caregiver when you look in the mirror, the sooner you're going to start taking care of number one.

■ Become an "expert." Knowledge is power. Learn as much as possible about the condition of the person you're caring for, how it will change over time, how change will affect care needs, and what to expect at the end of life. Not only will this make you a better caregiver, it will make you better able to communicate with the care recipient, the physician(s), and other health-care providers. A good source of information would be the physician(s) you're dealing with. Other good sources are local and national organizations devoted to specific conditions, such as the American Cancer Society, Alzheimer's Association, or American Heart Association. They can also connect you with local support groups. And a geriatrician is a good source of information if the care recipient has Alzheimer's disease, another form of dementia, or multiple conditions.

■ Reduce stress. Lighten up. Be realistic about what you can and can't do as a caregiver. (The Alcoholics Anonymous Serenity Prayer works for caregivers, too!) Identify problems and break them down into manageable steps. Learn to recognize the early warning signs of stress, and then make changes or adopt strategies that help lighten caregiver burden and responsibilities. Learn yoga or deep breathing exercises, and use them when you feel the stressometer ticking over into the red zone. And, to quote a former First Lady, "Just say no." This is one instance where it actually works.

■ Practice smart eating. As I stressed in Chapter 3, no matter what your age, you are what you eat. Make sure that your diet is well balanced and nutrient-dense, so that your body has what it needs (especially protein, micronutrients, and carbohydrates) to provide energy, make repairs, and protect against the physical and emotional strain of caregiving. Since your hectic schedule may not always allow you to eat when and what you should, take a high-potency multivitamin, too.

■ Exercise regularly. Don't give up your three nights a week at the gym, and if you don't have a workout routine, create one by working exercise into your daily routine. Do stretching and toning exercises before you get out of bed in the morning, walk up the six flights to your office, and use part of your lunch hour to power-walk. Regular physical activity helps reduce tension and depression, promotes better sleep, and boosts alertness, energy, and stamina.

■ Get proper rest. Studies show that people who don't get at least seven hours of sleep a night are prone to depression and accidents, and they're also more vulnerable to illnesses. If you can't get all the sleep you need at night, take a twenty- or thirty-minute nap. A study funded by the National Institute of Mental Health showed that a midday snooze could help reduce the effects – irritation, frustration, stress – of the emotional overload that comes with caregiving.

■ Practice preventive health care. The physical and emotional demands of caregiving don't just increase emotional stress; they have a direct and negative impact on your immune system and physical health. Don't skip your annual vaccinations, checkups, and visits to the dentist. See your doctor for little problems – back pain, tension headaches, exhaustion – before they become big ones. Join a support group or see a psychotherapist if your emotions seem to be controlling your actions, rather than the other way around. Talk therapy isn't just blowing off steam; it's a way to discover solutions to seemingly insurmountable problems.

■ Ask for and accept help. Trying to be all and do all for a loved one is a prescription for depression, burnout, and resentment, not only of the person you're caring for but of all the family members and friends who see what you're doing and don't offer to help. Create a carebook (or order one developed by a nurse, *The Carebook: A Workbook for Caregiver Peace of Mind*, by calling 503-760-5750), and involve other family members in caregiving.

While the brother who lives in Seattle and the sister who lives in Boston can't supply hands-on care, they can manage insurance paperwork, contribute toward the cost of an adult day-care program, and/or come to stay for a long weekend while you take a much-needed break. Make a list of chores that can be delegated, so that when family members ask, "Can I help?" you're ready to sign them up. And be proactive in seeking out community services and social-service agencies that can provide as-needed and long-term help. (*See Help for Caregivers Is Just a Phone Call Away, page 144.*)

■ Know when you need a break and take it. Whether caring for someone twenty-four hours a week or 24/7, every caregiver needs a break from the responsibilities of caregiving. Having back-up caregivers, such as friends, neighbors, paid home companions, or adult day-care centers, allows you to take a break and recharge your emotional and spiritual batteries.

Holding a family meeting

When a family member becomes seriously ill or disabled, the entire family is affected. Though one person may have accepted the role of primary caregiver (whether reluctantly or willingly), all the family members who want to, including the care recipient, should be involved in the planning and decision-making that go into providing the necessary care.

Family meetings take the coordination skills of a four-star general and the ego-massaging skills of a Hollywood agent, but they're worth the effort. They get everyone on the same page and talking the same language with regard to the family member's health condition, diagnosis and treatment goals, care plan, and probable prognosis. In addition, they're a good place for the primary caregiver to share his or her concerns about the physical strain, emotional stress, and financial burden he or she may be dealing with and to parcel out caregiving duties, tasks, and responsibilities to the family members best able to provide them or pay to have them provided.

When family meetings are well managed – and bringing in a trained counselor or facilitator to keep them focused and on task just about ensures that – participants come away from the meeting feeling not only that they have had their say but that the caregiving plan is "their" plan as well. Family members who'll be providing long-distance caregiving (an increasingly common occurrence in today's geographically dispersed families) should probably walk out of the meeting with a carebook, the notebook or three-ring binder containing copies of medical, legal, financial, and social-service information, as well as a record of which family member has agreed to do what.

While the initial meeting should definitely have everyone in the same room, follow-up meetings usually can be handled with conference calls followed by a letter or e-mail that gets everything down on paper.

Peering into the future

If you're a woman of 50 or older, odds are that you'll be taking on the care-giver role twice: for parents in their late 70s or 80s and for your spouse. If chronic health conditions are involved, caregiving may begin even earlier.

Knowing you'll be stepping into the caregiver role means that you have time now to plan for it. To begin planning, talk frankly with parents and your spouse about the future. That means discussing such subjects as finances and where important documents are stored, the type of housing that would best serve everyone's needs, the pros and cons of long-term-care insurance, and legal documents like a will or durable power of attorney for health care.

Long-Distance Caregiving

Your 79-year-old mother calls you at work from a hospital in Boston. She's been in a car accident. She's fine, she says, but both her legs are broken. She'll be in the hospital for a week and then will go to a skilled-nursing facility for six to eight weeks. She just thought you should know.

A panicky call to her physician gets you more information. "She rear-ended a car at a stoplight," he says. "I've been trying to get her to give up driving for more than a year."

That night you call and suggest – plead! – that Mom come to Cleveland and live with you. Your request is met with a frigid "I don't think so."

And just like that, you've become a long-distance caregiver.

Long-distance caregivers should download a free copy of *Handbook for Long-Distance Caregivers* (www.caregiver.org) and use the phone and the Internet to:

- **Gather information** – About Mom's medical condition; about her current and projected health-care needs; about services provided by your company's human resources or Employee Assistance Program; about the Family Medical Leave Act, which permits a person to keep his or her job while taking up to twelve weeks of unpaid leave to care for a family member; about people "on the ground" who can provide care and services; and about how these services can be paid for.

- **Put together a care team** – Of siblings and other family members; Mom's close friends and neighbors; professionals, such as the family physician and nurse, banker or financial planner, lawyer, handyman, or housekeeper who know Mom well; members of Mom's church or synagogue; members of organizations Mom belongs to; and volunteers from Faith in Action (877-324-8411 or www. fiavolunteers.org).

- **Create a three-ring-binder carebook** – With contact information for all the individuals listed above; contact information on local service providers, agencies, and home-care services; copies of financial and legal documents; and copies of the charts, lists, and check-off sheets from the Centers for Medicare and Medicaid Services (www.careplanner.org).

- **Contact a care manager/case manager** – to be responsible for the on-the-ground coordination and management of care and service delivery.

Also, think about the skills that might be needed on a caregiving team and who might best fill the bill.

Put together a folder that contains important medical and health-care information, including medications being taken, contact information for primary care physicians and specialists, insurance policy numbers, etc. This folder will come in handy if the person you're caring for is admitted to an emergency room, hospital, or skilled-nursing facility.

Research community-support services and agencies. If you know you're going to be providing care to someone with a specific disease or condition, you can obtain helpful information from the local organization addressing that disorder, including how to contact area support groups.

Start getting prepared for the emotional, ethical, and cultural struggle and power shift that comes with the role of caregiver.

Whoever first said, "Growing old isn't for sissies" wasn't alluding only to the aged. It's just as appropriate for caregivers.

Hiring a caregiver

As our population of older adults has expanded, the number of agencies that provide home companions and home-care aides has increased, and more individuals are offering in-home care as well.

Hospital-based services and reputable agencies can be found through the Yellow Pages, under Home Care or Home Health Services. Most offer their employees ongoing training, which increases their skill levels and marketability as well as the salaries they can command. In addition, the agencies do all the necessary background checks, drug screens, and employee bonding; employment paperwork (paychecks, with deductions for Social Security, Workers' Compensation, and employee health-care insurance); and scheduling to ensure that you have the help you need when you need it. All you have to do is call, outline your needs, interview a person or two, and sign up.

You also can hire an independent caregiver – usually at a rate that's significantly less per hour than you'd pay an agency. Best bets for finding good caregivers are friends, neighbors, or your clergy; the local senior center, social workers, and discharge planners at local hospitals or nursing homes; the local Area Agency on Aging; or the want ads.

If you go that route, be prepared to interview several applicants; collect the phone numbers of references and interview them about the applicant; contact an agency or private investigator (found in the Yellow Pages under Detective Agencies or Investigators) or Internet service (www.knowx.com, www.informus.com, and www.crimecheckinc.com are recommended by the National Alliance for Caregiving) to perform background checks; sign up as an employer with the Social Security Administration, the state Workers' Compensation department, and your city, county, and state taxing authorities; create and sign a contract with the in-home caregiver; and then be sure to supervise the caregiver's activities.

If you'll only be using a home-care aide a couple of times a month, it's probably smarter and less of a hassle to call an agency. If you're hiring someone full-time, however, you'll save money if you hire the aide and perform the supervision yourself.

Appendix 1
Myths and Realities of Aging

Simply put, because they've had so much more life experience, people over 65 are a far more diverse group than those under 25. Still, they are lumped together into an age "cohort" that has spawned hundreds of myths. Here are some of the most erroneous, along with the realities behind them.

Myth: *Genes determine longevity.*

Reality: While genes do play an important role in who will get diseases early in life, by the time people reach their late 40s, lifestyle and environmental factors play a far more crucial role in longevity.

Myth: *Chronological age is the true indicator of how "old" a person is.*

Reality: Chronological age indicates the passage of time; biological age indicates the wear and tear that's taken place in an individual's systems and organs. Many things – the use of antioxidants, exercise, not smoking – can slow biological aging.

Myth: *To be old is to be dependent.*

Reality: The percentage of people over the age of 65 living in nursing homes has been steadily declining and is currently around 5 percent of the population of those over 65. In their groundbreaking book *Successful Aging*, John Rowe, M.D., and Robert Kahn, Ph.D., found that a substantial majority of Americans between 75 and 84 reported no disability, and that even after age 85, four in ten reported they were fully functional.

Myth: *Ill health is an inevitable and immutable part of aging.*

Reality: Just as the percentage of those over 65 who are in nursing homes has gone down, so has the percentage of those in their late 60s, 70s, and 80s who are disabled by illness and disease.

Myth: *In old age, tooth loss is inevitable.*

Reality: Dental health status is not a result of age. It is the consequence of systemic diseases and inflammation, pharmacological interactions, functional disabilities, and cognitive decline. Treatments based on this information are saving teeth.

Myth: *Older people are resistant to change.*

Reality: A flexible attitude and the capacity to adapt to circumstances have more to do with lifelong personality than age, and long-term studies of those 65 and over have found little individual decline in people's intellectual sharpness, reasoning, and analytical ability until they reach their early 80s. And Rowe and Kahn reported in their book *Successful Aging* that with training, people could improve cognitive function and short-term memory. However, by age 85, about 50 percent of older people will show some signs of Alzheimer's disease.

Myth: *Older people can't master new information.*

Reality: Some loss of brain cells does occur with age, but it has little effect on brain function. Intellectual functions such as reasoning, vocabulary, and learned skills often improve with age. Crystallized intelligence or the ability to use accumulated knowledge to solve problems and make decisions increases throughout life. However, fluid intelligence, which is related to response time and recall, does decline.

Myth: *Memory loss is inevitable.*

Reality: While memory loss is not a normal part of aging, a slowing in the ability to recall recent information (i.e., recent memories) is common. Anxiety and depression, fatigue, stress and grief, adverse drug reactions, high fevers, and poor nutrition can temporarily affect memory. Alzheimer's disease, strokes, and long-term alcohol use are the major causes of irreversible memory loss.

Myth: *Age puts the kibosh on passion and romance.*

Reality: The need for affection, companionship, and sex does not change with age, so while sexual responses are slowed by factors related to aging (vaginal dryness, erectile dysfunction due to diabetes, arthritis), they are not eliminated. Those who had an enjoyable sex life before age 65 will continue along that path; conversely, those who did not will continue along *that* path.

Myth: *Aging is accompanied by urinary incontinence.*

Reality: While it is more common in those over 65 and those living in nursing homes, urinary incontinence is not a normal consequence of aging. With medications, lifestyle or behavior modification, and/or surgery, 80 percent of urinary incontinence can be significantly improved or cured.

Myth: *Personality changes with age.*

Reality: Unless the brain is affected by a medical condition such as Alzheimer's disease or stroke, personality patterns tend to persist throughout life. People who were gregarious or easygoing when they were younger will continue being so; the same is true if they were introverted or hypercritical.

Myth: *Older people require less sleep.*

Reality: It's not that they require less sleep, it's that they tend to get less. And the quality of the sleep they do get – especially the rapid-eye-movement (REM) sleep that is needed for physical restoration – is poor when sleep patterns are disrupted by daytime napping and frequent awakenings at night.

Myth: *Depression, loneliness, and grief are normal for older people.*

Reality: None of these feelings is more usual in late life than in early life. However, older people are faced with many situations that can bring them about, such as loss of a loved one, a severe medical condition, or a move to a nursing home. Therapies employing behavior modification and antidepressant medications are extremely successful, achieving an 80 percent rate of cure and/or symptom modification.

Myth: *Substance abuse is not common among the elderly.*

Reality: Unless treated at earlier stages, illegal drug and alcohol abuse follows people into old age; you don't see many older abusers, however, because they have died from abuse-related complications.

Myth: *There's little that older people can do to improve their health status.*

Reality: By the time you reach middle age, lifestyle is the major determiner of health and physical status, and it's never too late to change bad lifestyle habits. Stopping smoking, even at 60, can reduce the risk of cancer and heart disease. An exercise program begun at 65 will improve cardiovascular function (which lessens the chance of a stroke) and muscle strength (which lessens the chance of a fall that can lead to a nursing-home admission).

Appendix 2
Ten Natural Medicines That Will Improve Your Diet and Health

When Hippocrates, the father of Western medicine, said, "Let food be thy medicine and medicine thy food," he wasn't talking about turning food into pills and potions; he was imploring his patients to choose foods that enhanced their health and well-being along with filling their stomachs.

Today we know that the medicine he was talking about is the naturally occurring compounds found in foods. Besides the vitamins, minerals, and trace elements (such as boron, iodine, and zinc) necessary for building strong bodies, these compounds include antioxidants (compounds that corral the free oxygen radicals responsible for tissue destruction), phytochemicals (plant-derived compounds that have disease-fighting properties), and prebiotics and probiotics (compounds that promote intestinal health).

These compounds seem to boost the immune system's ability to fight germs and infections and/or delay or modify the severity of many of the symptoms and conditions associated with aging, including high blood pressure, heart disease, stroke, certain kinds of cancers, diabetes, bone and joint disorders, and vision-robbing macular degeneration and glaucoma.

You've been consuming natural medicine all your life; you just never thought of cholesterol-lowering garlic, gut-cleaning yogurt, or cavity-preventing tea as medicine.

While the biggest source of natural medicine is plants – and the less processed they are, the better – natural medicine is found in all foods. To boost the healing power of your diet, eat more of the following:

1. **Berries**. The USDA Human Nutrition Research Center on Aging recently found that dark-colored berries – blueberries, strawberries, etc. – contain extremely high levels of antioxidants.

2. **Brewer's yeast**. This supplement, which is available as a powder, flakes, or tablets, is an excellent source of high-quality protein and B vitamins, both of which become increasingly important as you age. (Too much, however, may cause nausea or diarrhea.)

3. **Crucifers**. Broccoli, cabbage, and all the other members of the huge crucifer clan are loaded with vitamins and minerals, fiber, and phytochemicals, including isothiocyanates, which studies suggest may protect against a variety of cancers.

4. **Fiber**. Dietary fiber – the indigestible skin, pulp, seeds, etc., left over when the nutrients have been extracted from fiber-dense fruits, vegetables, beans, and nuts – keeps the gut healthy. And it keeps gastrointestinal disorders, heart disease, obesity, and diabetes at bay. To increase fiber, add bran or psyllium seed husks to your diet.

5. **Fish**. Virtually all fish are sources of omega-3 fatty acids, which promote heart health. Eating unfried fish two or three times a week is associated with a low risk for heart disease. In addition, fish is an excellent source of high-quality, easily digested protein.

6. **Functional foods**.Invented by the Japanese, these are foods, such as calcium-fortified orange juice, that have had their nutritional content boosted with extra vitamins, minerals, or other compounds. Or they're products – such as the cholesterol-lowering margarine Benecol – created to address specific health issues.

7. **Nuts and seeds**. Yes, they're packed with calories, but they're also packed with energy, good fats and oils, protein, and fiber. Both nuts and seeds produce a feeling of fullness, so they make an excellent snack.

8. **Soy products**. Rich in calcium, minerals, and trace elements, protein, and plant estrogens, products made from soybeans boost immune function and may offer pre- and post-menopausal protection against osteoporosis.

9. **Tea**. All teas are rich in compounds called catechins, which research indicates may protect against heart disease, stroke, tooth decay, and certain cancers. And tea is a tasty way to meet some of your daily water requirement.

10. **Yogurt**. Fermented dairy products are excellent sources of calcium, protein, and vitamin B_{12}. Because they tend to promote gut health, they may also boost immune-system function and help reduce the risk of stomach and colon cancers.

Appendix 3
Resources for Caregivers

Books, Guides, and Directories:

Because We Care: A Guide for People Who Care. Administration on Aging (http://www.aoa.gov/prof/aoaprog/caregiver/carefam/taking_care_of_others/wecare/wecare_intro.asp)

The Carebook: A Workbook for Caregiver Peace of Mind. Joyce Beedle, R.N., B.S.N. LadybugPress, 1999 (This binder workbook is excellent for keeping track of the needs of care recipients. To order, call 503-760-5750.)

The Caregiver Helpbook: Powerful Tools for Caregiving. Vicki L. Schmall, Ph.D., Marilyn Cleland, R.N., Marilynn Sturdevant, R.N., M.S.W., L.C.S.W., Legacy Caregiver Services, 2000

Caregiver Resource Directory. http://www.netofcare.org/

Caring for the Parents Who Cared for You: What to Do When an Aging Parent Needs You. Dr. Kenneth P. Scileppi. Citadel Press, 1996

Caring for Yourself While Caring for Your Aging Parents: How to Help, How to Survive. Claire Berman. Henry Holt & Company, 2001

Changing Places: A Journey with My Parents into Their Old Age. Judy Kramer. Riverhead Books, 2000

The Comfort of Home: An Illustrated Step-by-Step Guide for Caregivers. Maria M. Meyer and Paula Derr. Care Trust Publications, 2002

The Complete Eldercare Planner: Where to Start, Which Questions to Ask, and How to Find Help. Joy Loverde. Three Rivers Press, 2000

The Complete Idiot's Guide to Caring for Aging Parents. Linda Colvin Rhodes, Ed. D. Alpha Books, 2001

Coping With Your Difficult Older Parent: A Guide for Stressed-out Children. Grace Lebow and Barbara Kane, with Irwin Lebow. HarperCollins, 1999

ElderCare 911: The Caregiver's Complete Handbook for Making Decisions. Susan Beerman and Judith Rappaport-Musson. Prometheus Books, 2002

Elder Care: A Six Step Guide to Balancing Work and Family. John Paul Marosy. Bringing Elder Care Home Publishing, 2000 (This is a workbook with many reproducible worksheets. To order, call 508-854-0431.)

Elder Rage, or Take My Father…Please!: How to Survive Caring for Aging Parents. Jacqueline Marcell. Impressive Press, 2001

Everyday Grace: Having Hope, Finding Forgiveness and Making Miracles. Marianne Williamson. Riverhead Books, 2002

How to Care for Aging Parents. Virginia Morris. Workman, 2004

It Takes More than Love: A Practical Guide to Taking Care of an Aging Adult. By Anita G. Beckerman, A.R.N.P., C.S., Ed.D., and Ruth M. Tappen, Ed.D., R.N., F.A.A.N. Health Professions Press, 2005

Loving Your Parents When They Can No Longer Love You. Terry Hargrave. Zondervan, 2005

The Memory Bible: An Innovative Strategy for Keeping Your Brain Young, Gary Small, M.D. Hyperion, 2003

Self-care for Caregivers: A Twelve Step Approach. Pat Samples, Diane Larsen, Martin Larsen, and Marvin Larsen. Hazelden, 2000

Successful Aging. J.W. Rowe, R.L. Kahn. Pantheon Books, 1998

Taking Care of Aging Family Members: A Practical Guide. Wendy Lustbader and Nancy Hooyman. The Free Press, 1994

Taking Care of Mom, Taking Care of Me: How to Manage with a Relative's Illness and Death. Sima Devorah Schloss. The Judaica Press, 2002

There's a Spiritual Solution to Every Problem, Wayne Dyer. HarperCollins, 2001

The 36-hour Day: A Family Guide to Caring for Persons with Alzheimer Disease, Related Dementing Illnesses, and Memory Loss in Later Life. Nancy Mace and Peter Rabins, M.D., M.P.H. Warner Books, 2006

When Bad Things Happen to Good People, H.A. Kushner. Avon Books, 1997

Organizations

Administration on Aging . . . . .www.aoa.gov

Alzheimer's Association . . . . .www.alz.org

American Association of Homes and Services for the Aging . .www.aahsa.org

Eldercare Locator . . . . .www.eldercare.gov

Family Caregiver Alliance . . . . .www.caregiver.org

Children of Aging Parents www.CAPS4caregivers.org

Individual State Caregiver Programs . . . .
www.aoa.gov/prof/aoaprog/caregiver/careprof/state_by_state/state_by_statepf.asp

National Academy of Elder Law Attorneys . . . . .www.naela.org

National Adult Day Services Association . . . . www.nadsa.org

National Alliance for Caregiving . . . . .www.caregiving.org

National Association of Area Agencies on Aging www.n4a.org

National Association of Geriatric Care Managers . . .www.caremanager.org

National Family Caregivers Association . . . . .www.nfcacares.org

National Family Caregiver Support Program . . . .
. . . . .http://www.aoa.gov/prof/aoaprog/caregiver/carefam/carefam.asp

Well Spouse Foundation . . . . .www.wellspouse.org

Health information resources

Cleveland Clinic Health Information Center . .www.clevelandclinic.org/health

Health Compass . . . . .www.healthcompass.org

Healthfinder . . . . .www.healthfinder.gov

Medicare . . . . .www.medicare.gov

Medlineplus Health Topics . .www.nlm.nih.gov.medlineplushealthtopics.htm.

National Organization for Rare Diseases . . . . .www.rarediseases.org

Senior Citizens' Resources . . . . .www.seniors.gov

Index

Other Books from Cleveland Clinic Press

Arthritis: A Cleveland Clinic Guide

Autopsy – Learning from the Dead: A Cleveland Clinic Guide

Battling the Beast Within: Success in Living with Adversity
  (about multiple sclerosis)

Breastless in the City: A Young Woman's Story of Love, Loss, and Breast Cancer

Forever Home (a chapter book for young readers)

Getting a Good Night's Sleep: A Cleveland Clinic Guide

The Granny-Nanny: A Guide for Parents and Grandparents
  Who Share Child Care

Heart Attack: A Cleveland Clinic Guide

Heroes with a Thousand Faces: True Stories of People with Facial Deformities
and their Quest for Acceptance

Overcoming Infertility: A Cleveland Clinic Guide

Planting the Roses: A Cancer Survivor's Story (about esophageal cancer)

Sober Celebrations: Lively Entertaining Without the Spirits
  (alcohol-free entertaining)

Stop Smoking Now! The Rewarding Journey to a Smoke-Free Life

Thyroid Disorders: A Cleveland Clinic Guide

To Act As A Unit: The Story of the Cleveland Clinic (Fourth Edition)

**Books are available from your local bookstore or from
Amazon.com and BN.com**

Cleveland Clinic Press

Cleveland Clinic Press is a full-line publisher of non-fiction trade books and other media for the medical, health, nutrition, cookbook, and exercise markets.

It is the mission of the Press to increase the health literacy of the American public and to dispel myths and misinformation about medicine, health care, and treatment. Our authors include leading authorities from the Cleveland Clinic as well as a diverse list of experts drawn from medical and health institutions whose research and treatment breakthroughs have helped countless people.

Each Cleveland Clinic Guide provides the health-care consumer with the highest quality, practical, useful, reliable, and authoritative information. Every book is reviewed for accuracy and timeliness by the experts of the Cleveland Clinic.

www.clevelandclinicpress.org

Cleveland Clinic

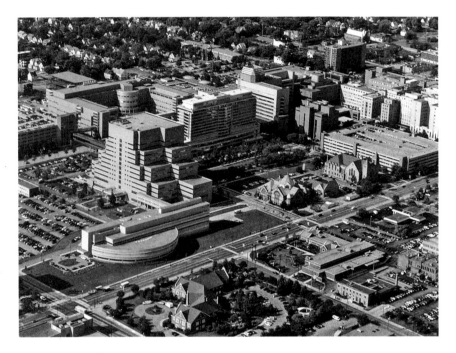

Cleveland Clinic, located in Cleveland, Ohio, is a not-for-profit multi-specialty academic medical center that integrates clinical and hospital care with research and education. Cleveland Clinic was founded in 1921 by four renowned physicians with a vision of providing outstanding patient care based upon the principles of cooperation, compassion, and innovation. *U.S. News & World Report* consistently names Cleveland Clinic as one of the nation's best hospitals in its annual "America's Best Hospitals" survey. Approximately 1,500 full-time salaried physicians at Cleveland Clinic and Cleveland Clinic Florida represent more than 120 medical specialties and subspecialties. In 2006, patients came for treatment from every state and 100 countries.

www.clevelandclinic.org